AF835900

COPING WITH DIABETES

JAN 1985

Other TAB Books by the Author

1804 *Coping with Your Bad Back*
1824 *Coping with Miscarriage*

COPING WITH DIABETES

BY OTHNIEL J. SEIDEN, M.D.

TAB BOOKS Inc.
BLUE RIDGE SUMMIT, PA. 17214

Notices

Tes-Tape is a registered trademark of Lilly.
Diastix is a registered trademark of the Ames Division of Miles Laboratories, Inc.
Clinitest is a registered trademark of the Ames Division of Miles Laboratories, Inc.
Chemstrip bG is a registered trademark of Bio Dynamics.

Illustrations by Anita Kay.

616.462
Sei
c1

FIRST EDITION

FIRST PRINTING

Copyright © 1984 by Othniel J. Seiden, M.D.

Printed in the United States of America

Reproduction or publication of the content in any manner, without express permission of the publisher, is prohibited. No liability is assumed with respect to the use of the information herein.

Library of Congress Cataloging in Publication Data

Seiden, Othniel J.
Coping with diabetes.

Includes index.
1. Diabetes. I. Title.
RC660.S39 1984 616.4'62 84-8898
ISBN 0-8306-1814-7 (pbk.)

Contents

Dedicated to Jack Charlier, a good friend who has beat diabetes.

Introduction

DIABETES IS A DISEASE, A DISEASE THAT TO THIS DAY IS INCURable. That does not mean, however, that it is a disease without hope. Indeed, the great majority of diabetics can live a very normal active, productive life, full of achievements, and capable of parenting normal, healthy families. Most diabetics who have come to grips with their disease will tell anyone, "Diabetes is the best incurable disease anyone could hope to have." There are diabetics who will tell you, "My diabetes is a blessing in disguise. If I wasn't a diabetic, I wouldn't be in the good shape and health that I'm in now!" No one is saying that people who don't have diabetes are missing out, but that statement is, in a way, the crux of coping with diabetes.

In a great majority of cases, the diabetic who takes care of himself and keeps his diabetes under control can live as normal, full, and exciting a life as anyone. There are exceptions, but thankfully they are a small percentage.

It is the purpose of this book to help you understand and cope with your diabetes, or that of your loved one or friend. The more you know about the disease, the easier it will be to cope.

It has been estimated that over 11 million Americans are diabetic. Possibly as many as half of them do not know they have the disease. There is a steady increase in the number of diabetics diagnosed every year, a figure approaching ¾ million. Though it is a disease that can in most cases be well controlled, 300,000 Americans die of it yearly. It is difficult to say where it belongs among the most common killers in our country. With 300,000 deaths a year, it is about fourth—behind cancer, heart disease, and stroke—except that it is often contributory to deaths listed in the statistics as heart disease, stroke, or renal failure. This disease costs our nation about 7 billion dollars each year for treatment and loss of production. These are gloomy facts, but they needn't be. Again I must emphasize that the great majority of diabetics who take care of themselves and control their diseases will not be among those who make up the bad statistics that give diabetes its bad image.

1: What is Diabetes?

DIABETES IS AN ANCIENT DISEASE. ANCIENT GREEKS NAMED it; the word diabetes means *siphon*. They recognized its most common and striking symptom: thirst. Patients have a seemingly unquenchable thirst when their disease is not under control. A second sign was also noted by physicians of old. The urine of diabetic patients attracted an inordinate number of flies and other insects because of the high sugar content. Thus, a Latin word *mellitus*, meaning honey, was added to the disease name. Most people discover they have diabetes mellitus not because they have any symptoms of the disease but because excessive sugar is discovered in their urine or blood during routine examinations.

Diabetes mellitus is usually classified into two major types: juvenile and adult-onset.

JUVENILE DIABETES

Only about 10 to 15 percent of all diabetics are what we classify as juvenile, or *insulin-dependent*, diabetics. Since insulin is destroyed when taken by mouth it can only be taken by injection. The juvenile diabetic is a member of that minority of patients who must take insulin shots, usually on a daily basis. Virtually all diabetic children have this type of diabetes, hence the name, juvenile. On the other hand, it is rare for a patient who develops diabetes in his adult years to have insulin-dependent diabetes.

Boys and girls are equally prone to juvenile diabetes. Diabetes

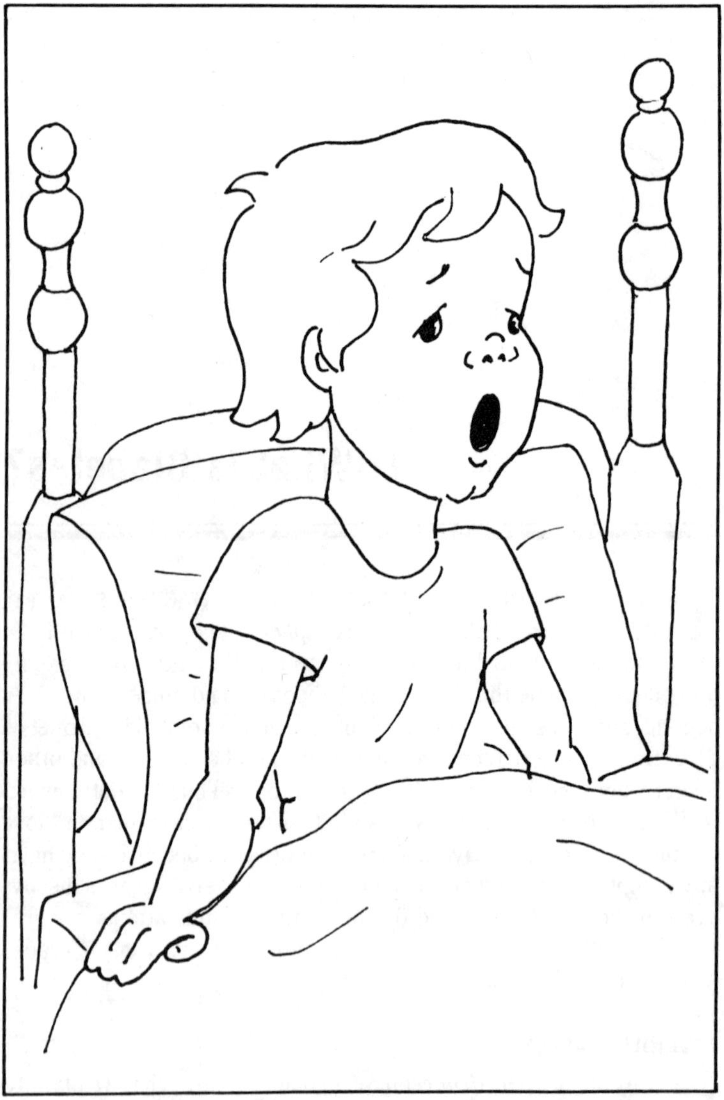

Fig. 1-1. There are many reasons why a child may begin to wet the bed again even after several years; diabetes must be considered as one of those possibilities.

which first appears during the teen years is also likely to be the insulin-dependent type. Diabetes with teenage-onset is frequently triggered by a severe infection or viral disease. It may be masked at first by the signs and symptoms of the triggering disease process.

This does not mean diabetes is caused by another disease, but more likely that the physical stresses of the triggering illness cause the latent diabetes to surface and become overt. Latent diabetes is a covert disease, with signs and symptoms undetected due to their mildness or absence.

The symptoms of juvenile diabetes vary, but commonly the following will be present:

Excessive Urination. Excessive urination is often the first clue to the onset of diabetes (Fig. 1-1). A child or teenager who suddenly begins to wet the bed after having had no such trouble should be checked for diabetes. Too often these children and teenagers are considered to have emotional problems, when it is elevated blood sugar and urine sugar which are causing the problem. It is not a matter of frequent urination of small amounts as in genito-

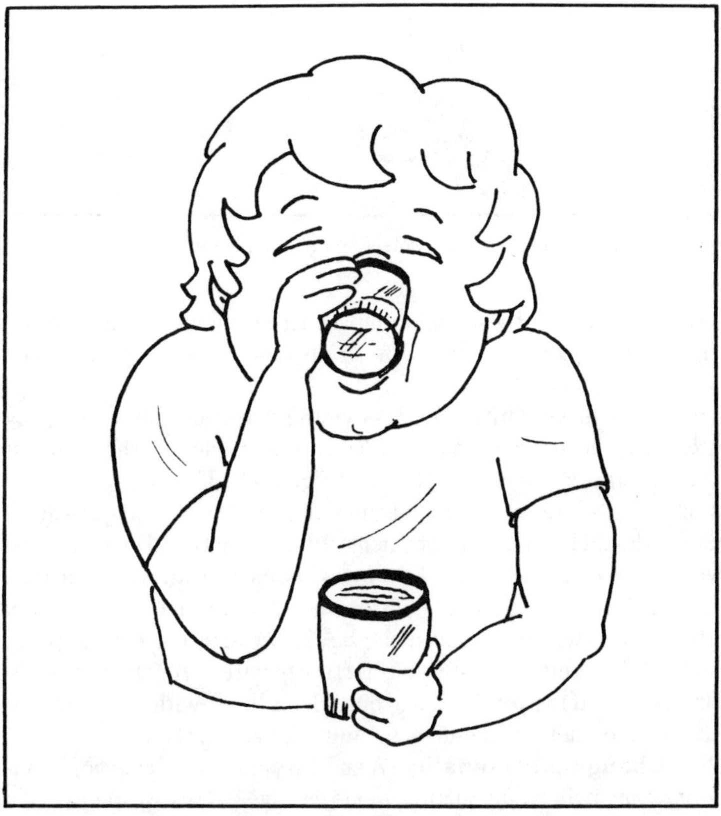

Fig. 1-2. Constant thirst for large quantities of water or other liquids is often an early sign of diabetes.

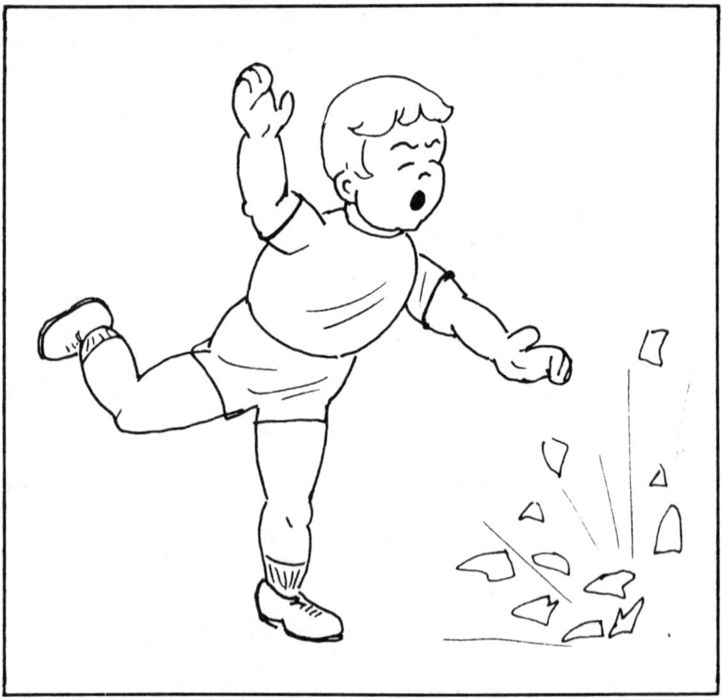

Fig. 1-3. Diabetes can bring on violent and abrupt personality changes.

urinary infection; these children pass large amounts of urine many times throughout the day. The urine may have an uncommonly sweet odor to it also.

Excessive Thirst. Excessive thirst will usually accompany excessive urination because the body must replenish the fluid lost through the kidneys and bladder (Fig. 1-2). The youngster who drinks glass after glass of fluid and still seems unable to quench his thirst should be taken to a physician for examination. Do not panic if your child or teenager drinks a few glasses of water or other fluid after he's eaten a bowl of chili or played vigorously and sweated profusely. The things that make us thirsty also make youngsters thirsty. The kind of thirst I am referring to here is constant throughout the day. If the youth tries to quench his thirst with sweet drinks, the development of the disease might be accelerated.

Changing Personality. A sudden personality change, irritability, and wildly fluctuating mood changes, loss of energy and interest, as well as dramatic changes in school work and grades, all might be signs of the onset of juvenile diabetes (Fig. 1-3). Of course these emotional changes are not too uncommon in children and especially teens, but they usually don't all occur at once. If they are accompanied by excessive urination and thirst, have the child examined.

Weight Loss. Weight loss is uncommon in a healthy child, as is the failure to gain (Fig. 1-4). Onset of juvenile diabetes frequently

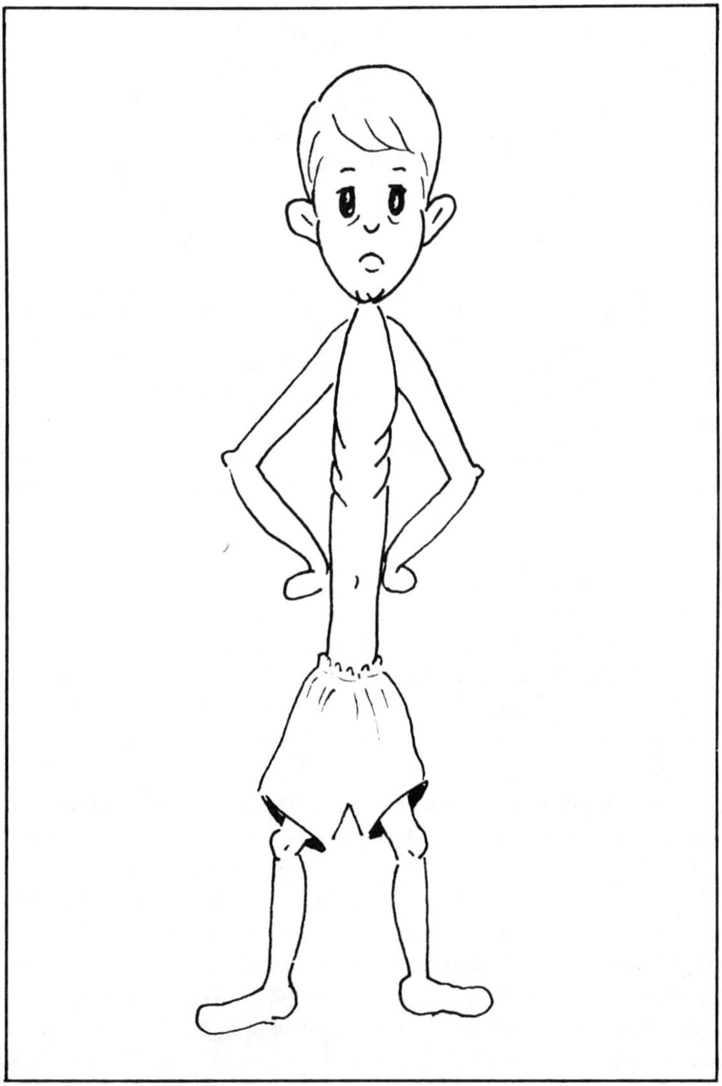

Fig. 1-4. Both weight loss and failure to gain can be indications of diabetes.

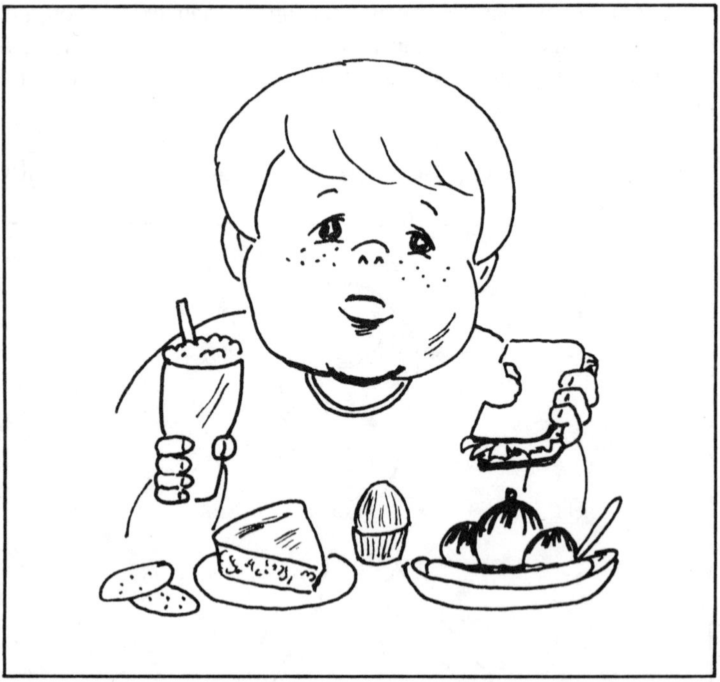

Fig. 1-5. A sudden or gradual enormous increase in appetite might be a sign of diabetes onset.

causes the retarding of growth and weight gain. Weight loss is even more of an indication that all is not right.

Insatiable Hunger. Even though the child or teenager may not be gaining or growing, or even losing weight, he may have a seemingly insatiable hunger (Fig. 1-5). If he selects lots of sweets and is constantly nibbling and eating, his diabetic condition may be accelerated.

Drowsiness. Drowsiness and coma are very late signs and symptoms of juvenile insulin-dependent diabetes mellitus (Fig. 1-6). It is rare for all the other signs and symptoms to be missed before coma occurs, but occasionally it does happen that the diagnosis is made after a child comes into a hospital or doctor's office in a coma. Usually this is a result of a severe flu, virus, or other infectious illness which puts an inordinate physical stress on the child's body. When a patient is difficult or impossible to rouse from deep sleep, coma must be suspected. Get medical aid immediately. Coma is usually preceded by rapid breathing, nausea, sleepiness and a pungent, acrid odor to the breath, known as *ketone breath*.

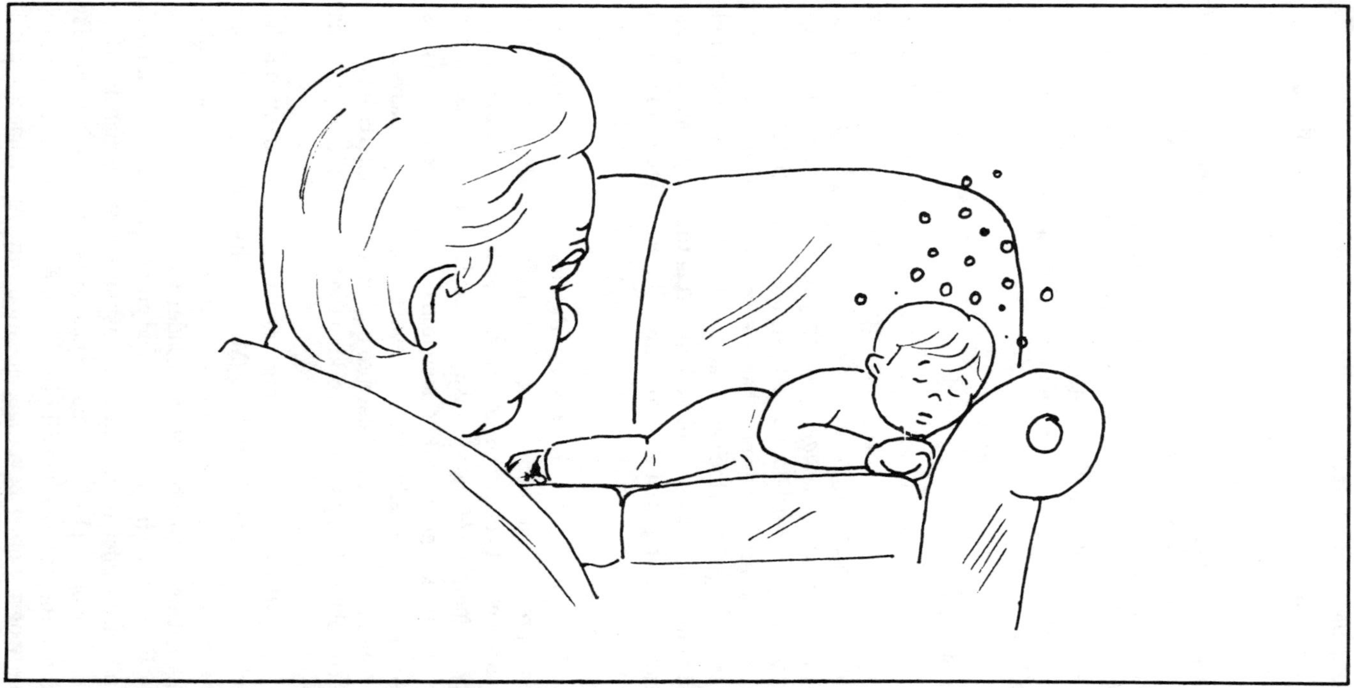

Fig. 1-6. Difficulty in rousing a patient is a very late sign of diabetes and may lead to coma.

ADULT-ONSET DIABETES

By far the most common type of diabetes is adult- or *maturity-onset* diabetes. About 85 percent of all diabetics are this type. They are able to produce some insulin themselves, but not enough to use all the sugar in their system, expecially if they are loaded with excessive carbohydrates due to a faulty diet. This form of non-insulin-dependent diabetes mellitus usually does not have its onset until middle age. Unlike juvenile diabetes which strikes boys and girls about equally, maturity-onset diabetes affects more women than men. Coma in this form of diabetes is very rare.

Symptoms

Symptoms of adult-onset diabetes mellitus are not as dramatic as those of juvenile diabetics and are easily overlooked for a long time because of their gradual onset. There is the old triad, *Polidipsia, poliuria, and poliphagia,* which physicians point out as presumptive signs of diabetes. Polidipsia is excessive thirst, poliuria is excessive urination, and poliphagia is excessive hunger. When they all appear together in the same patient, diabetes must be suspected. Most often the disease is picked up during routine physical examinations or during treatment for other illnesses. The following are some of the telltale warning signs that warrant further investigation:

Fatigue. Fatigue is probably the first and single most commonly present symptom of adult-onset diabetes (Fig. 1-7). Since the body gets its energy from sugar, and adequate insulin is necessary to metabolize blood sugar, it stands to reason that lack of energy and fatigue would be among the earliest signs of this disease. It is a sign easily missed, however, because it is easy to say, "I'm just not as young as I used to be," when we approach midlife, we complain, "I've just been working too hard," and let it go at that for a long time.

Urination. Urination at night is also a common symptom that is blamed on aging (Fig. 1-8). Most adults can sleep the night through or have to get up once in a while at most. The adult who must get up frequently should wonder why.

Constant Thirst. Constant and growing thirst to keep up with urinary frequency is another clue, just as in juvenile diabetes (Fig. 1-9). A lot of people do not realize just how much they drink in a day because they drink relatively little water. If you drink coffee constantly or any other beverage, question why. An undiagnosed dia-

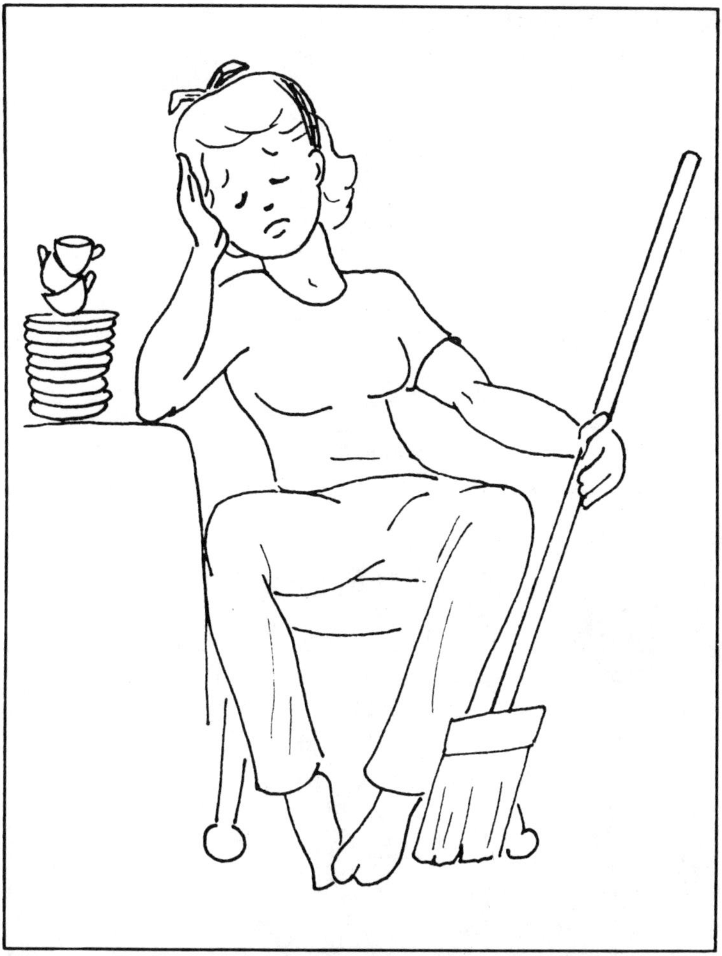

Fig. 1-7. Excessive fatigue is probably the first and single most common symptom of adult-onset diabetes.

betic may be drinking every 15 to 30 minutes and not even realize it. He goes to the bathroom almost as frequently and blames it on, "all that coffee I drink," and doesn't consider either as abnormal.

Weight Loss. Weight loss in the obese without dieting is a very unusual situation, except where adult-onset diabetes or other disease processes are concerned (Fig. 1-10). Adult-type diabetics are usually overweight; yet they sometimes have an onset of spontaneous weight loss before discovery of their diabetes.

Skin Infections. Skin infections are common among diabetics

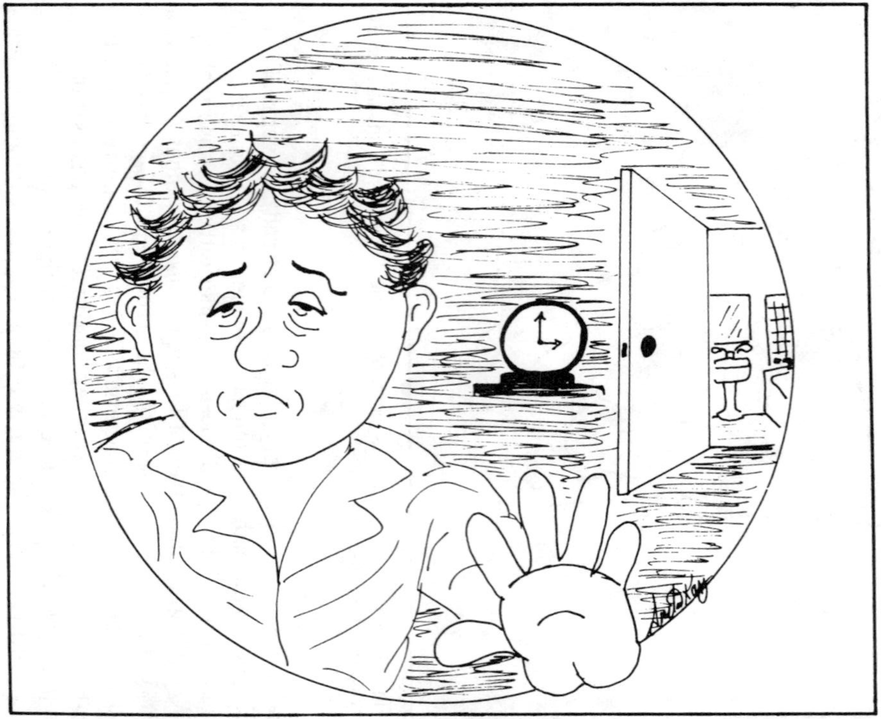

Fig. 1-8. Frequent and excessive urination may be the first noticeable sign of adult-onset diabetes.

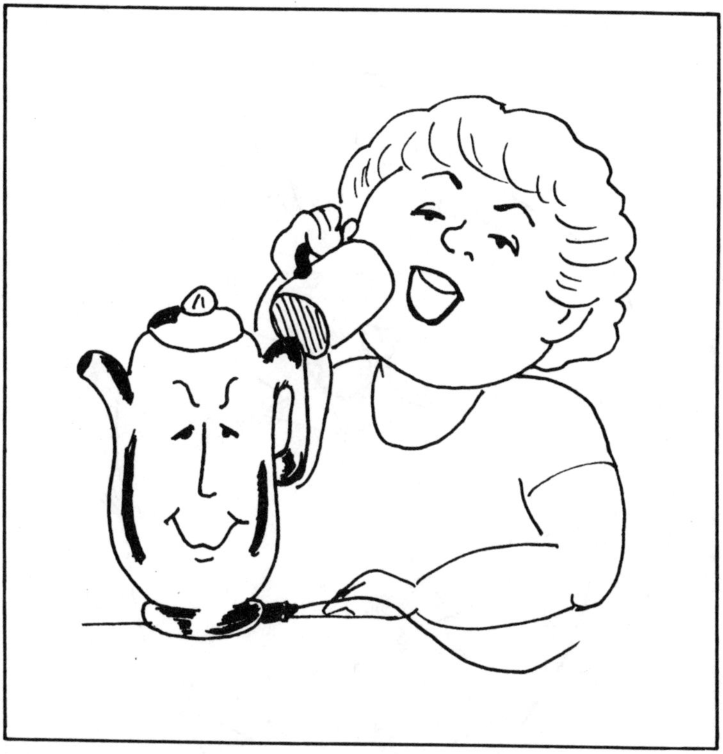

Fig. 1-9. As with the juvenile, adult-onset diabetes is accompanied by an enormous thirst.

whose blood sugar levels are too high. Boils, pimples, rashes, and eruptions are a direct result of the excessive sugar circulating in the blood, and they will improve as soon as the problem is brought under control (Fig. 1-11).

Visual Problems. Visual problems are also common in diabetics with too high blood sugars. The complaint is usually of blurred vision when changing one's view between objects of varying distances (Fig. 1-12). When blood sugar is markedly elevated, the lenses of the eyes tend to swell and will not change accommodation as rapidly as necessary. Because of this a person will notice some blurriness for a period of time when changing his gaze from something distant to an object nearby, or vice versa. This problem will resolve itself as soon as the diabetes is brought under control.

Neurological Changes. Neurological changes are among the late problems of adult-onset diabetes and indicate that the blood sugar has been drastically elevated for a long time. Numbness,

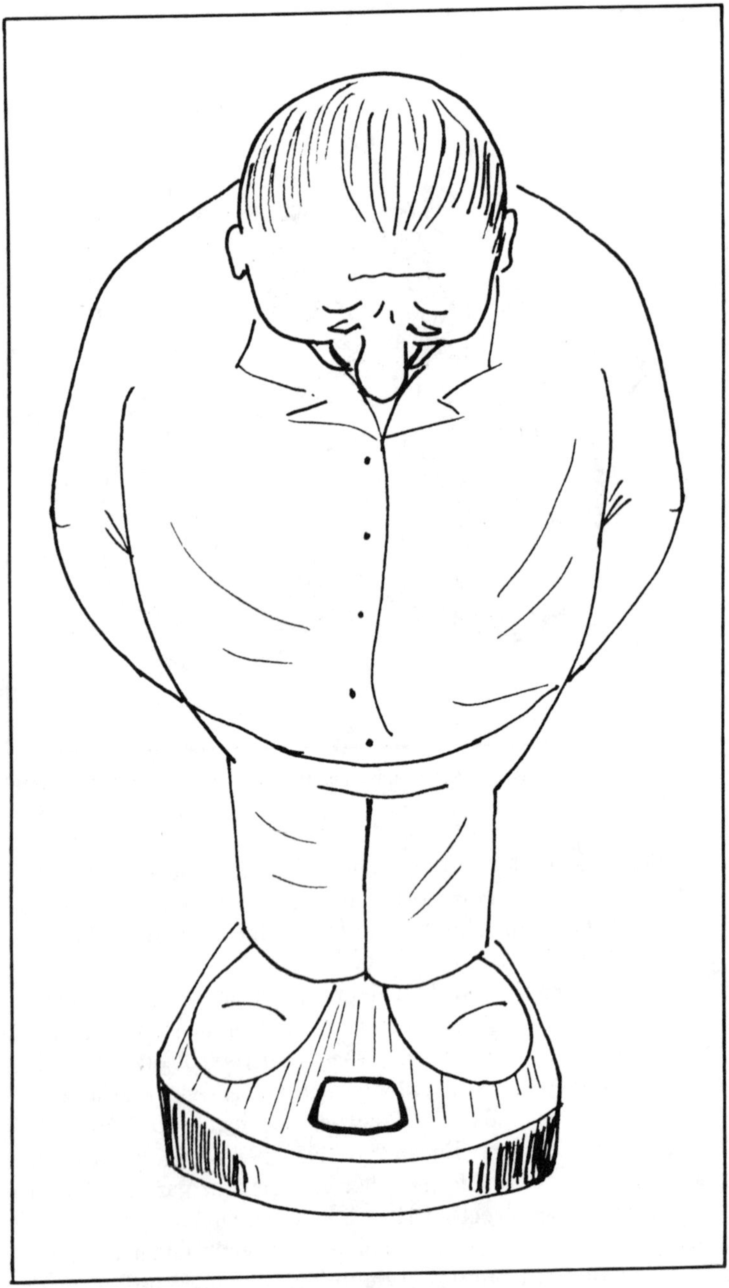

Fig. 1-10. Spontaneous weight loss without reduction in diet or increase in activity must be questioned.

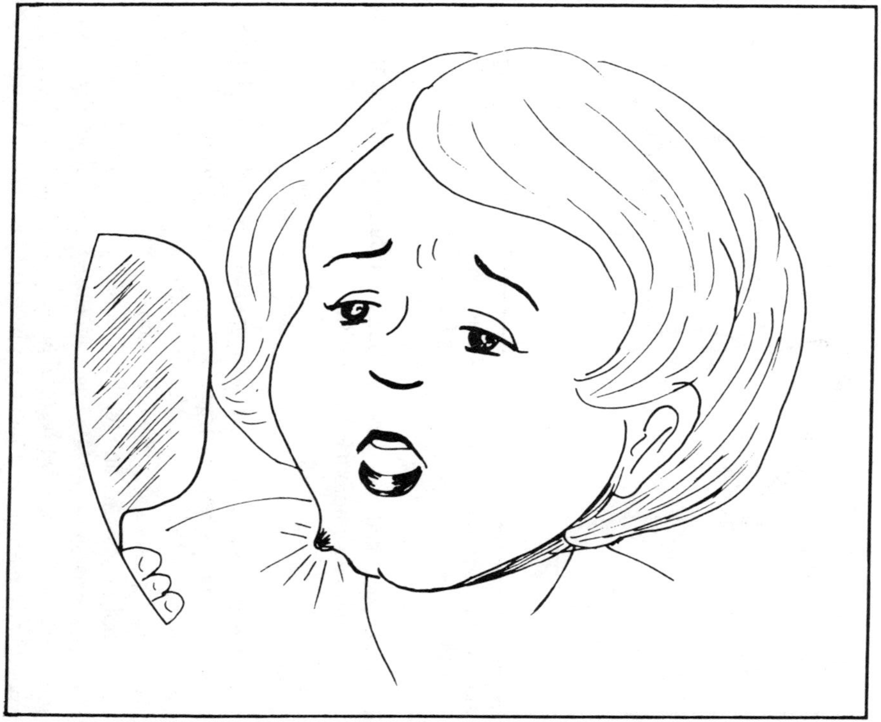

Fig. 1-11. Boils, pimples, and other complexion problems may indicate an abnormal elevation in blood sugar.

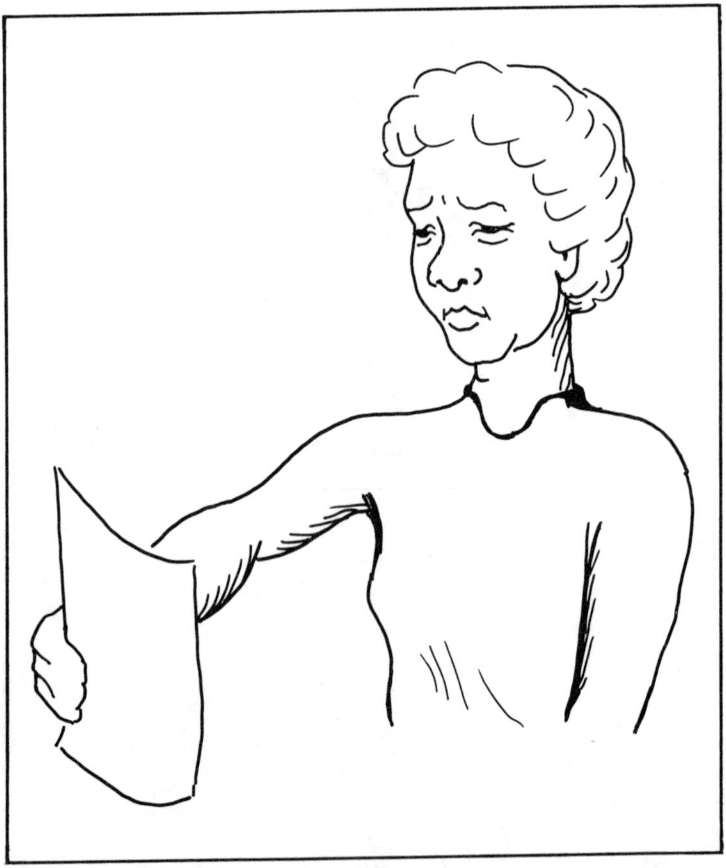

Fig. 1-12. Blurred vision, especially if it is intermittent, may be a sign that diabetes is present.

tingling, pain, and weaknesses usually in the extremities are the most common symptoms (Fig. 1-13).

Tests

Elevated sugar in either blood or urine laboratory specimens is by far the most common first clue that a person might have adult-onset diabetes (Fig. 1-14). Usually these tests are done as part of the routine screening in physical examinations. Elevation in a single test is not diagnostic, and further laboratory tests must be done. If one of the screening tests is positive, the doctor will usually order a glucose tolerance test with serial urine tests. The patient is given a specifically measured amount of glucose to drink, and then blood

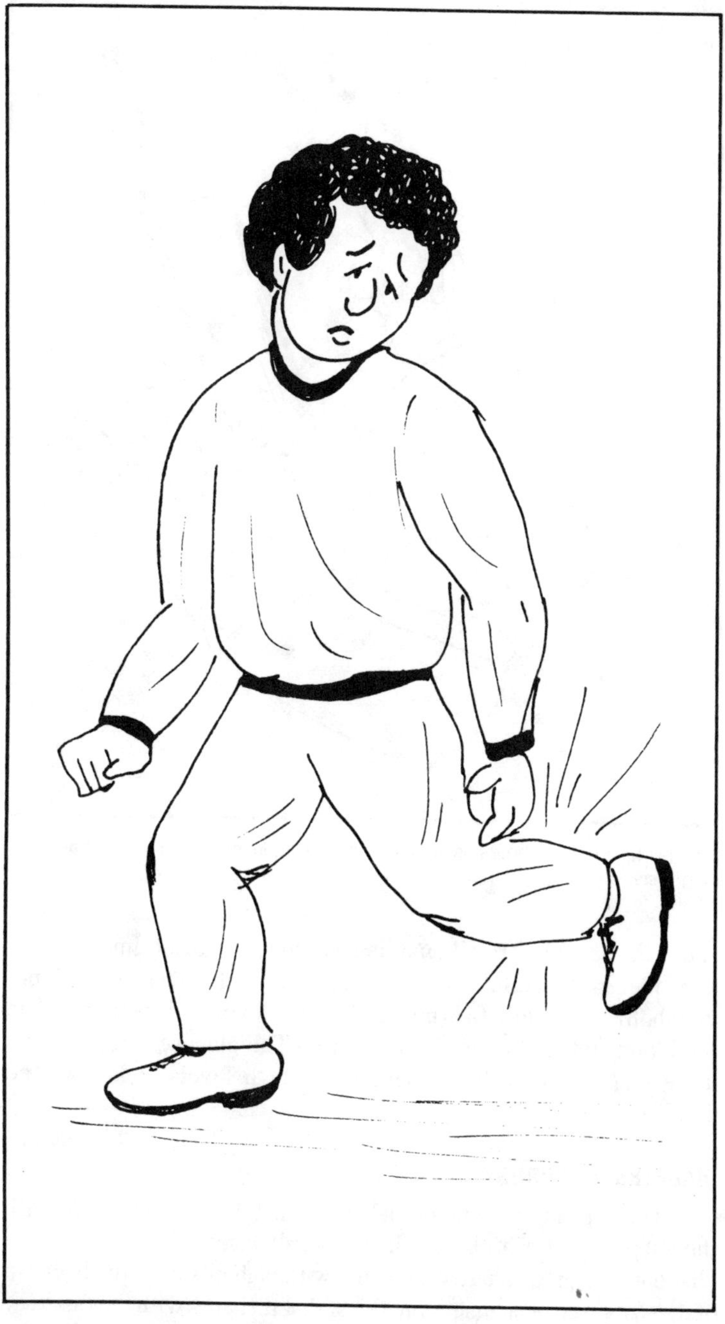

Fig. 1-13. Muscle cramping after limited activity must be treated with suspicion.

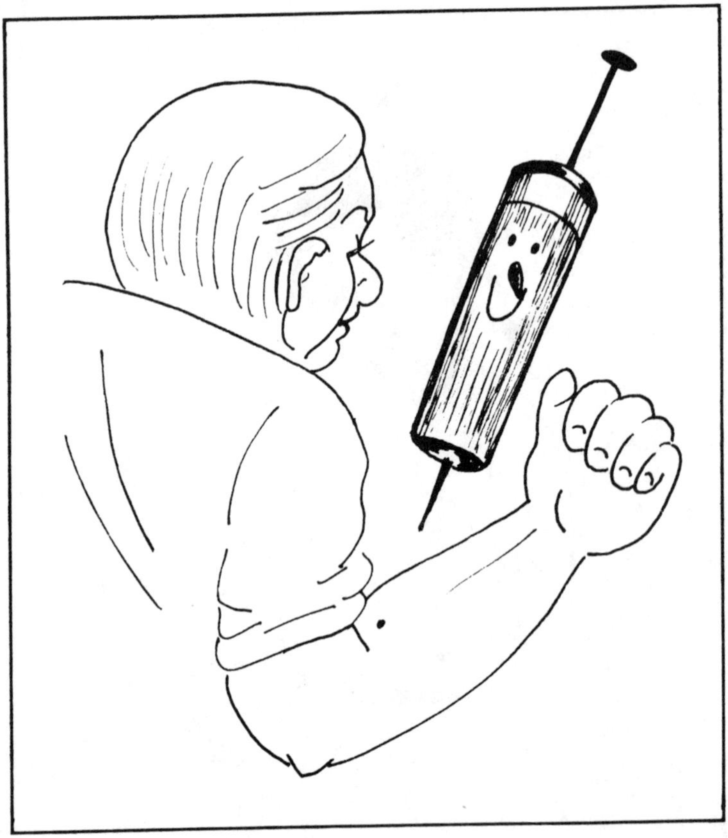

Fig. 1-14. When diabetes is suspected, a simple blood test can make the diagnosis.

and urine samples are taken at measured intervals of time. If there is inadequate insulin in the system, the blood sugar will not metabolize as rapidly as is normal, and the levels will remain high in the blood and spill over into the urine. The glucose tolerance and urine sugar tests will measure these high levels and make the diagnosis.

DIABETES INSIPIDUS

There is a third type of diabetes which has nothing to do with the subject matter of this book and is only briefly mentioned here. Diabetes Insipidus shares the name with diabetes mellitus because of the symptom of an insatiable thirst that it shares with the disease. Thus the similar name. It is rare, caused by a problem in the pituitary gland. It has nothing to do with sugar metabolism, insulin, or diabetes mellitus.

CAUSES OF DIABETES MELLITUS

What causes diabetes? Is it hereditary? Can you catch it? Who is most likely to get diabetes? These are common questions asked by patients or their loved ones.

Diabetes occurs when certain cells of the pancreas, located behind the stomach, stop producing sufficient insulin to regulate the metabolism of sugar in the body. These special cells that produce insulin are called *beta cells.* There are numerous reasons why these cells might malfunction or not function.

Heredity plays a part in the disease in certain cases. Diabetes does run in families, and if even one parent has the disease, the incidence in the children is considerably higher than in the general population. This does not mean that if a parent has the disease, all children of that parent will be diabetic, nor does it mean that a person is ensured of not getting diabetes just because no one else in the family has the disease.

Diabetes can also be caused by the destruction of the beta cells. There have been cases where disease or injury has required surgical removal of the pancreas and thus all of the beta cells. These patients are rendered diabetic and will have to take insulin shots for the rest of their lives.

In most cases the process that damages the beta cells is never known. People develop the disease in later life and no precipitating factor is ever detected. There is no preexisting virus or illness, such as often triggers juvenile diabetes. Many physicians feel that there is a yet undiscovered virus to which beta cells are sensitive. Other physicians feel that only beta cells predisposed by heredity are susceptible to viruses.

It is a well-known fact that excessive alcohol ingestion destroys beta cells along with other parts of the pancreas (Fig. 1-15). The incidence of diabetes among alcoholics is very high compared to the general public. In some cases even a small use of alcohol has been attributed with the onset of *pancreatitis*, a fulminating inflammation of the pancreas, and the precipitation of diabetes.

Diabetes is not considered a contagious disease. You could be couped up with diabetics all your life, and you would not catch the disease. There have been epidemics of flu, mumps, and other viruses which went through communities and were followed by a high incidence of newly diagnosed cases of juvenile diabetes after the epidemics, but in those cases the viruses seemed to trigger the onset of diabetes. There has never been an epidemic of diabetes.

Who is most likely to get diabetes? Less than 20 percent of all cases of diabetes occur before the age of 50. It is mostly a disease of the elderly. It occurs more commonly among the overweight population. Women are more prone to develop diabetes than men; the reason for this is not clear, but it is 50 percent more common in women. Certain races seem to have a higher incidence of diabetes; the American Indians have a very high incidence of the disease. Also the disease tends to appear much more frequently in the poor, which may well be from dietary and activity factors.

Diabetes is often discovered during pregnancy (Fig. 1-16). Dietary changes and the stresses of pregnancy seem to precipitate the disease in some who are predisposed. If a diabetic expectant mother takes care of herself under the supervision of a competent

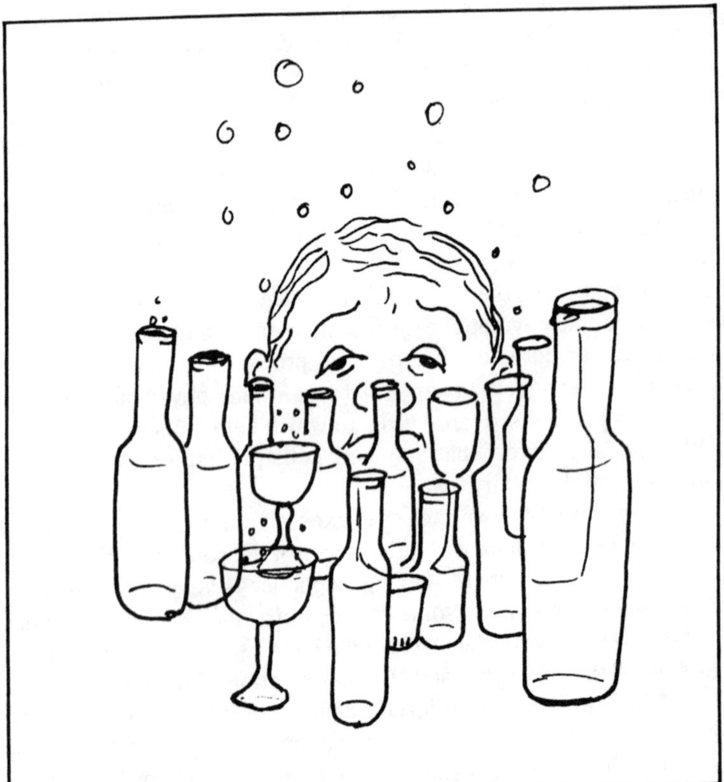

Fig. 1-15. Alcohol ingestion can precipitate and even cause diabetes.

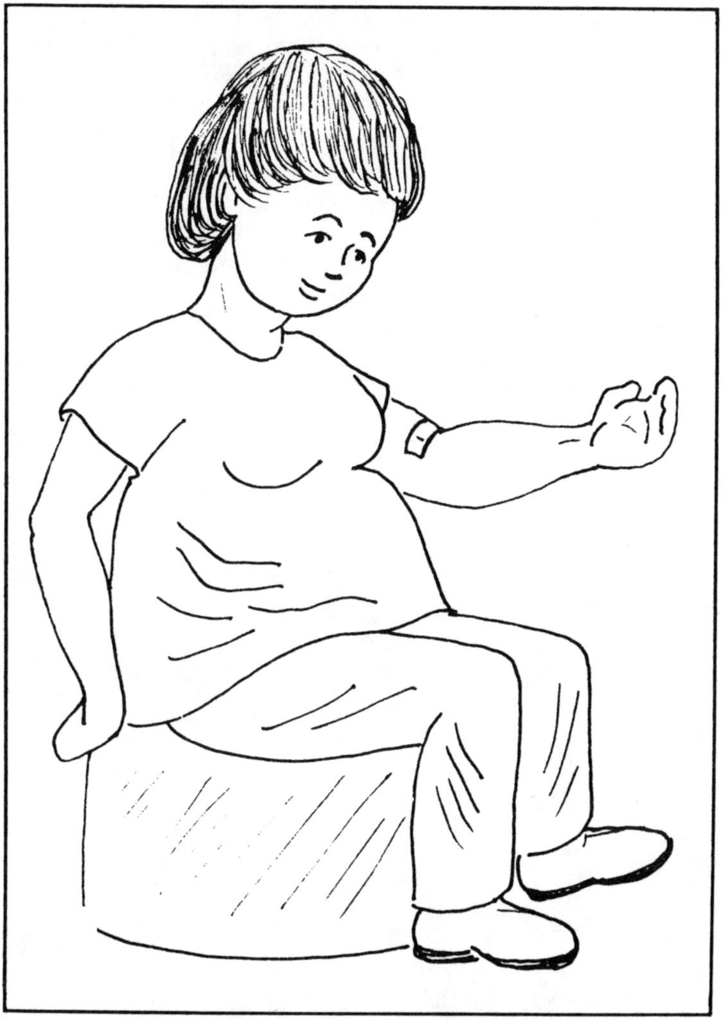

Fig. 1-16. Diabetes is often discovered during pregnancy.

physician during her pregnancy, she will probably deliver a healthy, normal baby without harm to her own health. After the delivery, her diabetes may go into remission and not reappear until her middle age or during subsequent pregnancies. If there is diabetes in the family, the physician should be told about it anytime there is a pregnancy or illness among any member of the family.

2: Treatment: Cure or Control?

THE TREATMENT OF DIABETES IS AIMED AT CONTROL, NOT cure. To date there is no cure for diabetes. If your body is unable to produce insulin, it must be replaced by injection. If your body is able to manufacture small amounts of insulin, then control is achieved by balancing the amount of insulin with the amount that can be provided. *Control*—that is what treatment of diabetes means. Once control is achieved and maintained, your disease is no longer a threat to your life and well-being. Your diabetes is being successfully treated. It is that balance between insulin need and insulin availability for which treatment is aimed.

This balance is achieved by controlling three factors in your life; your diet, your body's insulin supply, and your activity level. At worst this may be a nuisance to you, at best, a blessing, since controlling your diabetes will improve and maintain your general fitness at a higher level than the general public will ever attain. Whether it is a nuisance or a blessing for you will depend mainly on your attitude.

Let's approach these three basic factors of your treatment—insulin supply, diet, and activity—one at a time.

INSULIN

What is insulin? How does it work? What does it do?

Insulin is a chemical produced by the beta cells of the pancreas that acts as a catalyst in the conversion of blood sugar into usable energy by the cells of the body. Actually, insulin makes it possible for circulating sugar, which in the blood is in the form of glucose, to pass through the walls of the body cells where it can be used. It is as if the membrane that surrounds a living cell had a lock on it to keep out glucose. Insulin is the key to that lock. Without sufficient insulin to open the barrier, the blood sugar cannot get into the cell where it can be utilized. Without glucose, cells cannot function; if deprived long enough, cell death will occur.

In addition to making the cell walls penetrable by glucose, insulin stimulates, or *catalyzes*, the conversion of glucose into usable energy in all cells of the body.

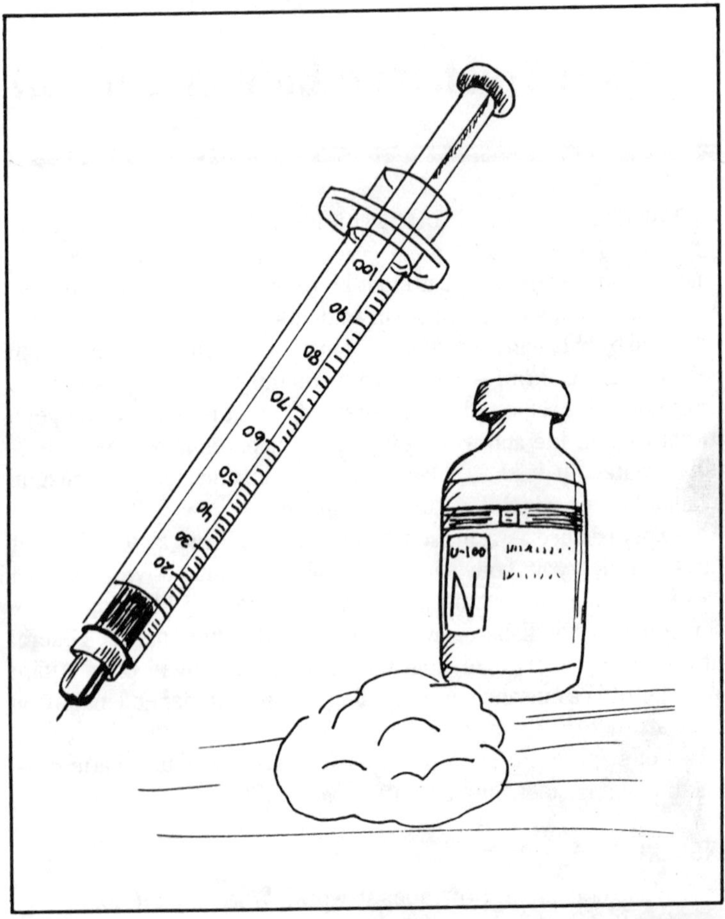

Fig. 2-1. The diabetic may require painless injections of insulin to control his or her disease.

Insulin also regulates the storage of unused sugars by catalyzing the conversion of glucose into storage fat which is then deposited for later use.

It becomes obvious that if your body cannot furnish sufficient insulin to maintain all its necessary functions something must be done to bring diet, activity, and insulin supply back into balance. One way to do this is to replace the insulin which is missing through medications (Fig. 2-1).

The most well-known medication for the treatment of diabetes is injectable insulin. It would surprise most people to discover that only a small percentage of all diabetics require insulin injections. Virtually all juvenile diabetics must inject themselves with insulin on a daily schedule, but remember, only a small percentage, under 15 percent, of all diabetics are juvenile types.

There are several types of injectable insulin. Determining the type and dosage that is best for you is the responsibility of your physician. It may take some time to work out the best medication program for you. Each person's requirements are different. Two things will help bring about the proper program for you in the shortest possible time:

- Be totally honest with your physician when he asks you about your habits and lifestyle.
- Follow his instructions to the letter and let him know when you have had to deviate from his instructions.

He cannot be expected to balance your diet, medication, and activity if you alter the variables or ground rules without his knowledge.

Insulin Types

Regular Insulin. Regular insulin, or soluble insulin as it is usually called outside the United States, is a fast but short-acting insulin. It is a pure form which does not have protein or zinc additives to prolong its effectiveness. Your physician will prescribe it if your lifestyle and diet demand a quick onset of insulin action for short duration. Regular insulin starts to work on your blood sugar in about 30 minutes after injection and has its peak action in 2 to 3 hours. It is spent in about 5 to 6 hours. Patients who use regular insulin exclusively may have to inject themselves several times a day.

NPH Insulin. NPH insulin, usually called Isophane insulin outside the United States, is, on the other hand, a slow-onset, longer-acting medication. It does not begin to function until 2 to 3 hours after injection. Its peak action is about 8 to 16 hours after injection, and it is not fully spent for up to 24 hours. This is ideal for patients who are active and away from home, so they do not have to inject themselves during the day. There must be considerable regularity to their diet and activity from day to day so that insulin need can be predicted and balance maintained over long periods of time.

Lente Insulin. Lente insulin is very similar to NPH and shares similar characteristics.

Semilente Insulin. Semilente insulin, on the other hand, is similar to regular, or soluble, insulin. It has a rapid onset but a slightly longer duration of action—up to 4 or 5 hours.

PZI and Ultralente Insulin. Ultralente insulin and PZI (protamine-zinc insulin) are very long-acting insulins. Their onset of action may begin a little slower than NPH and Lente insulins, and their peak actions will span from 9 to 24 or more hours depending on the patient's metabolism level. PZI and Ultralente insulins may not be fully spent from the body for up to 36 hours.

Dosages of Insulin

All these types of insulin are obtained from the pancreas of cows and pigs and are usually a mixture of both beef and pork insulin. Pure beef and pork insulins are available. Some patients are sensitive to beef insulin, others must avoid pork because of religious dictates.

In the United States, insulin is made available in 100 unit dosages, called U-100 insulin. It used to be available in U-40 and U-80 dosages and still is outside the United States. U-100 means that there are 100 units of insulin in a cubic centimeter or milliliter of injectable fluid.

If you are among the small percentage of diabetics who must use insulin, the type and dosage your physician will prescribe for you will depend on both your usual diet and lifestyle (Fig. 2-2). The more varied these variables are, the more difficult balancing your insulin will be. Patients who can maintain a very regular diet and activity level can usually use the longer-acting insulins, thus requiring less frequent injection (Fig. 2-3).

Above all you must never change your insulin type, dosage, or schedule without your physician's knowledge or supervision. Some patients who must take insulin feel a deep resentment to their situation and consciously or subconsciously rebel against taking

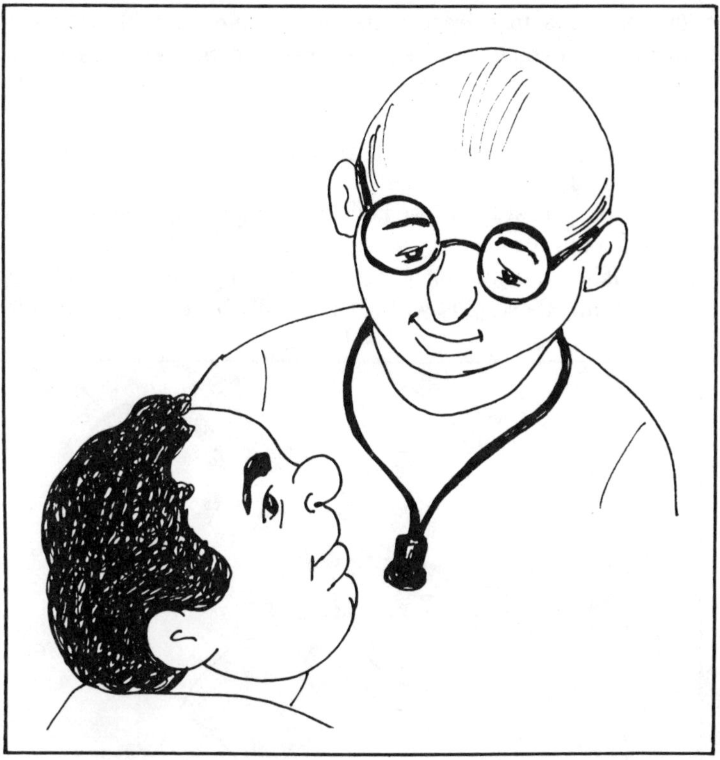

Fig. 2-2. Control of diabetes is a team effort between patient and doctor.

their medication as prescribed. It is important that you make your feelings understood to your physician so that he can help you work out your hostilities. It is important to your future well-being. You should make yourself understand that you are fortunate to be living in an age where insulin is available to you. Before 1921 this life-saving medication was unavailable to insulin-dependent diabetics, and their activities and lives were drastically limited and shortened.

ANTIDIABETIC PILLS

In recent years antidiabetic pills have come into use. These oral medications are helpful to some adult-onset diabetics (Fig. 2-4). Antidiabetic pills are not an oral form of insulin! They cannot replace insulin injections for the juvenile or insulin-dependent diabetic!

Oral hypoglycemic agents, another name for antidiabetic pills, lower your blood sugar in two ways. First, they act as a stimulant to your pancreas to release more insulin into your blood stream. Obviously, if you are a juvenile or insulin-dependent diabetic, and your pancreas cannot produce insulin, it cannot be stimulated to release the substance. Second, they reduce the amount of insulin needed by your body by making your body's cells more sensitive to the reduced insulin available.

Also, it must be pointed out that oral hypoglycemics will not help all adult-, or maturity-onset diabetics. If you are considerably overweight, or if your blood sugar runs consistently over 300 mg. per 100 ml., these pills will not markedly benefit you. The ideal

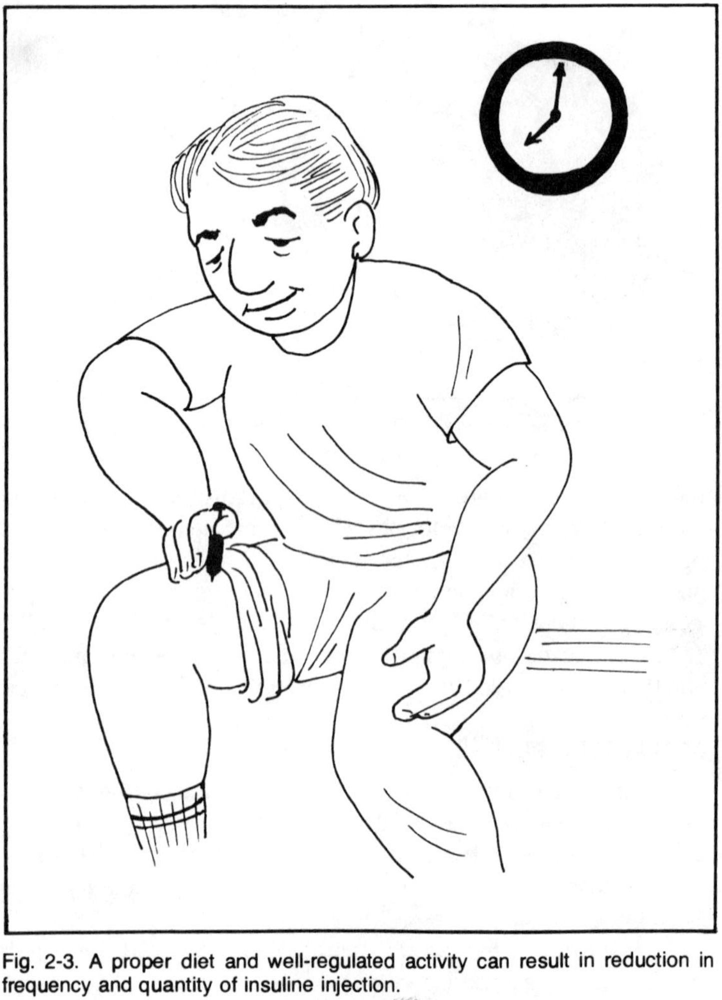

Fig. 2-3. A proper diet and well-regulated activity can result in reduction in frequency and quantity of insuline injection.

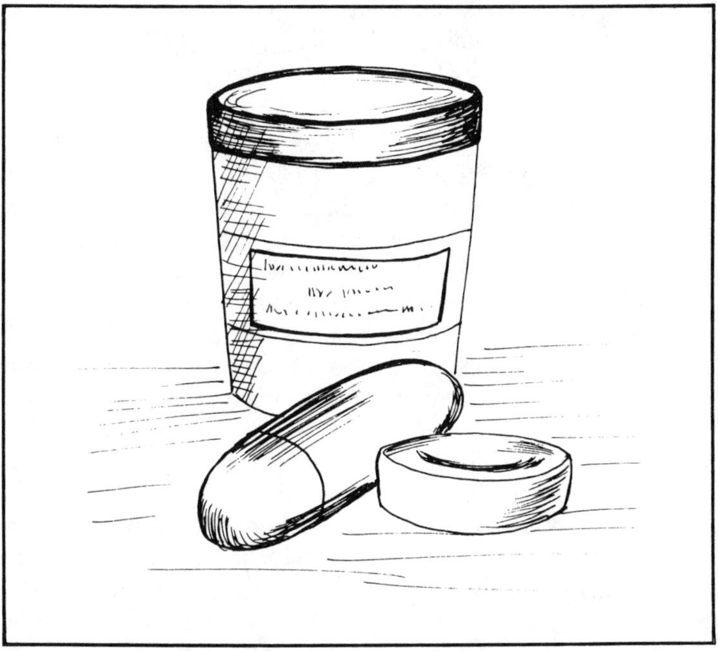

Fig. 2-4. Many adult-onset diabetics can control their diabetes with oral medication.

candidate for use of oral hypoglycemics is an adult with mild diabetes who is lean and still runs a blood sugar up to 200 mg. per 100 ml. despite regulation of diet and moderate activity. If diet and activity will not bring your blood sugar below 200 mg. percent, then you may be among the few adult-onset diabetics who must occasionally use insulin injection.

Besides not working for everyone who is diabetic, oral hypoglycemics have some other unfavorable side effects which bear consideration. You should be aware of them. The following symptoms are not usually serious, but should be immediately called to the attention of your physician when noticed:

- Diarrhea
- Nausea
- Heartburn and stomach discomfort
- Loss of appetite
- Headache

These symptoms will usually disappear when the pills are discontinued, or the dosage is adjusted. More serious but much more rare are the following side effects:

- Unusual, persistent, and severe fatigue
- Dark urine, similar to the color of strong tea or cola
- Sore throat and fever
- Unusual bruising or bleeding
- Yellow coloration of the whites of the eyes and/or skin

A dispute has raged since 1970 as to whether or not oral hypoglycemics increase the incidence of death by heart attack. Evidence is still inconclusive. Studies have supported both sides of the argument. My view is that if the oral hypoglycemics are used in the right patients—those who will benefit from them—their advantages far outweigh the disadvantages. The person to determine if you should use the oral hypoglycemic pills is your physician. Discuss them with him fully and understand why he decides for or against their use in your case. If he prescribes them for you, it is important that you use them with confidence. Anxiety and stress over their use may be counterproductive.

Once more let me emphasize the great majority of diabetics will be able to control their disease with diet and activity alone. If they do have to resort to the use of medication, either oral or injective, it will probably be of short duration, perhaps during periods of stress, illness, pregnancy, or lifestyle change.

DIET

For the great majority of diabetics diet is the key to balancing blood sugar. The adult-onset diabetic who can keep his or her weight in reasonable limits and can maintain a moderate and regular activity level will probably never need to use medication. The juvenile diabetic who can maintain a balanced diet and activity level will have a minimum problem with insulin getting by with a minimum dosage and injection schedule.

Much has changed in the basic philosophy of diabetic diet design in recent years. Diabetic diets of old contained a lot of fat and protein with the exclusion of as much sugar, fiber, and carbohydrate as possible.

Carbohydrates

The main source of carbohydrate foods is plants. Carbohydrate is one of our most important sources of body energy; so to eliminate it from the diabetic diet, as was practiced in the past, is a disadvantage. Two types of carbohydrates exist in nature: sugars and starches. The grains, such as wheat, rice, potatoes, barley, oats,

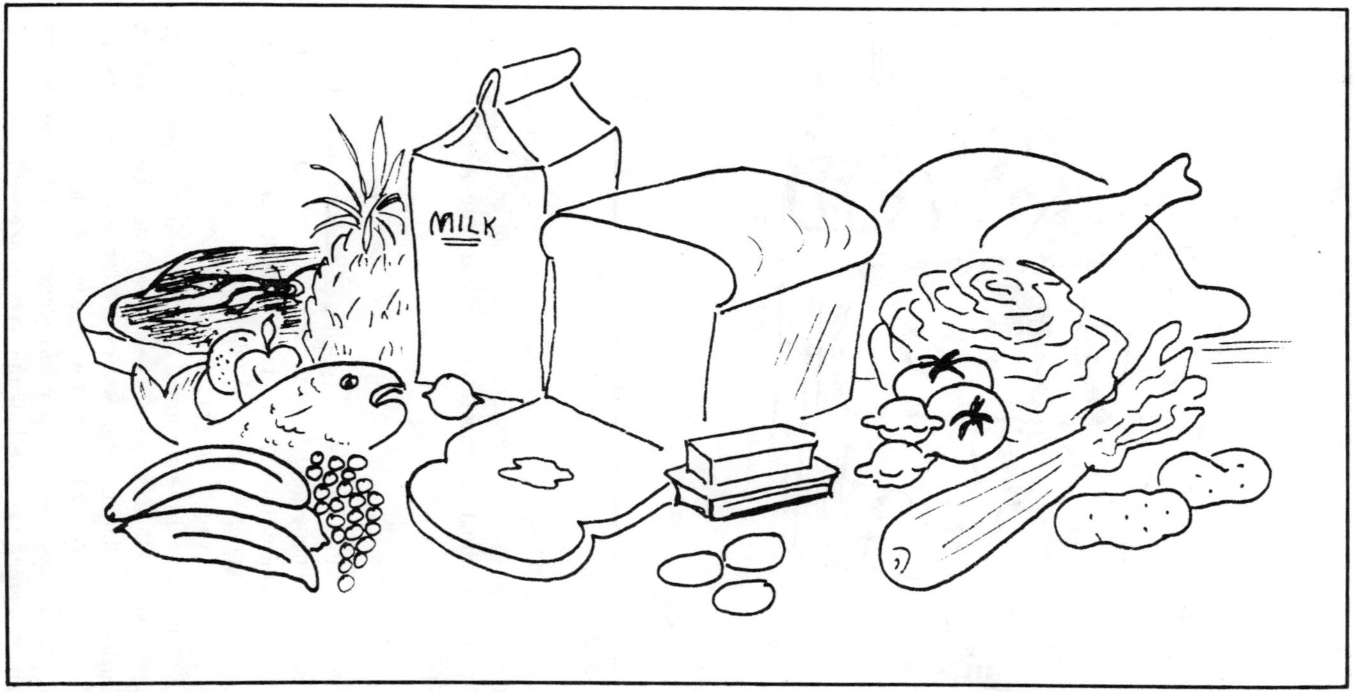

Fig. 2-8. Vitamins.

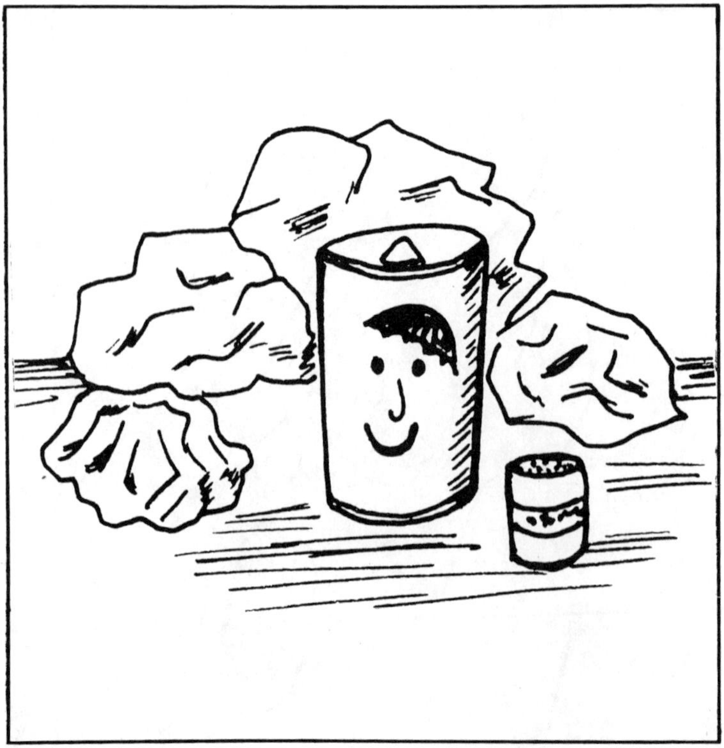

Fig. 2-9. Minerals.

chain (Fig. 2-9). Again, the need for these trace elements is no greater for the diabetic, although deficiency in both vitamins and minerals might affect the diabetic quicker and more overtly than the nondiabetic.

Fiber

Another name for fiber is roughage. Fiber is not a nutrient perse, but is nonetheless vital to our diets and well-being. Roughage increases the bulk of our diet without increasing calories. It is provided by the undigestable "skeleton" or shells and husks or outer coating of vegetation (Fig. 2-10).

Often this valuable portion of the vegetable foods we eat has been thrown away. In the past, when wheat was ground into flour, the husks, or shell, of the grain was most often discarded. The same was true of rice. Whole rice or brown rice was shelled and made into white rice. This increased the caloric content per volume that we ate and discarded valuable bulk our system needed.

Now whole-grain cereals, rices, and breads have come into their own. The person who eats brown rice will get far fewer calories per volume of food than the person who eats white rice, and the food will be better for him. Some grains have as much as 60 percent fiber. To discard their fiber content actually can double their caloric content per volume eaten.

Not only is whole-grain food lower in caloric content, but because it is less processed, it contains far more of its original vitamin and mineral values. Whole-grain foods aid tremendously in proper digestion. Roughage also absorbs water and sugar in the intestines, binding it and reducing its absorption into the blood, thus helping to lower blood sugar and keep insulin requirements down. Roughage helps the body maintain regular bowel function and elimination of waste material. The person who eats sufficient fiber will have little need for laxatives. In addition there is growing evidence that high-fiber diets reduce the incidence of diabetes, stroke, heart disease, obesity, and colon cancer.

Diabetic Diet of the Past

In the past, diabetic diets consisted of maximum elimination of

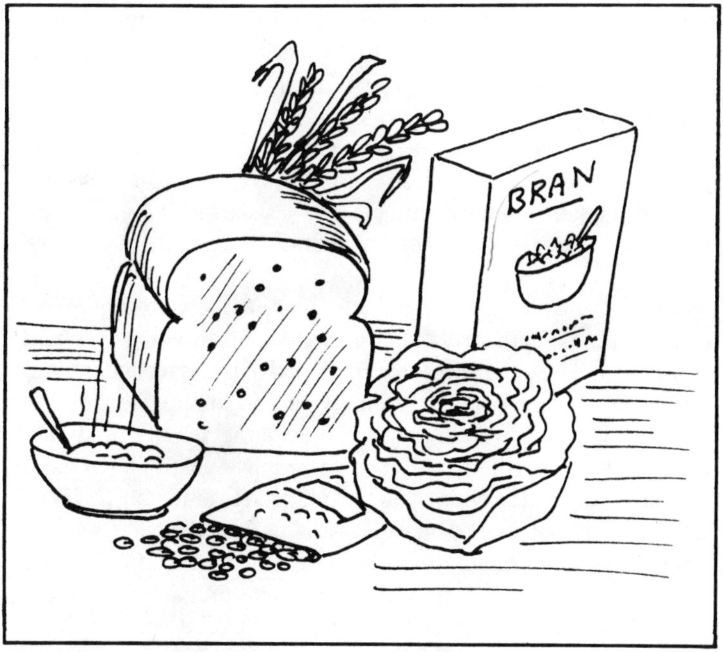

Fig. 2-10. Fiber and roughage.

starch and carbohydrates and an emphasis on protein and fat. The idea stemmed from the logical conclusion that, since insulin was needed to metabolize sugar, the lack of adequate insulin made it important to eliminate sugar from the diet. Starch was also eliminated because it was nothing more than a complex sugar. Fat was emphasized in diabetic diets as an energy source to take the place of sugar. Protein was given in high quantity because meats were also an excellent source of fat, and protein affected the blood sugar less than other foods.

It was a theory that held for centuries, but not because there was scientific evidence to back it. It was theory put into practice and never tested. As a result, diabetics have had high blood cholesterols and high incidences of hardening of the arteries, heart disease, and stroke. It was then noted that many diabetics who refused to follow the unpalatable strict diabetic diets of old, did quite well and didn't have the high morbidity and mortality from circulatory diseases.

At last "dogma" about traditional diet was put aside for scientific research into the best kind of diet for diabetics. In 1976 the results of some of this research was published in the *American Journal of Clinical Nutrition*. The article introduced the "High-Carbohydrate, High-Fiber" diet (the HCF diet). Actually, the HCF diet is not only for the diabetic; its principles and benefits apply to the nondiabetic as well. We all benefit from lowering our blood cholesterol and absorption of sugars. Though all diabetics seem to benefit from HCF diets, the best results are with adult-onset types.

A word of caution: do not alter your diet on your own. Your physician should make all decisions in the treatment of your diabetes. If you do not have faith in the job he is doing, change physicians, but do not try to control your diabetes without the care of a competent physician.

It is not in the scope of this book to prescribe your diet. Your specific diet must come from your doctor or a nutritionist to whom he refers you. The purpose of this section is to help you understand the principles behind your diet. Simply put, by adding fiber to your diet, your digestive system helps to reduce the amount of fat and sugar absorbed into the blood. You will probably be able to eat a more varied diet and reduce your insulin requirements. You may lose weight without strict denial of food. This does not mean you can eat sugars and carbohydrates at will. Even nondiabetics should reduce their sugar intake drastically. You will probably be able to moderately increase your starch intake. Your diet must still be carefully balanced by your physician to your individual needs.

ACTIVITY

The third phase in controlling your diabetes is activity. Activity includes all the energy spent, or calories burned, in your work, leisure, and exercise time. The most important aspects of your activity are: that it is sufficient to balance your diet and insulin levels, and that it is regular. It will be virtually impossible for your physician to balance your blood sugar if your energy expenditures are erratic from day to day. Vigorous activity and exercise are vital to everyone's health, all the more so to the diabetic.

Vigorous activity, of course, is necessary to keep you fit: to maintain good muscle tone, strength, and endurance; to keep your cardiovascular system in top performing shape, and to keep your vital organs functioning to maintain general good health. Regular activity is necessary to maintain a reasonably constant expenditure of energy each day (Fig. 2-11). A controlled exercise period each day is the easiest and best way to manage both regular and vigorous activity.

There is no activity that the diabetic cannot do because of his or her diabetes. Other physical limitations might prevent you from taking part in a particular sport or activity, but not your diabetes, unless it has already affected other organs of your body, such as your cardiovascular system. There are diabetics among Olympic athletes, high school and college stars, professional athletes in all sports—football, baseball, skating, skiing, tennis, golf, you name it. Your diabetes should not stand in the way of any achievement you want to attain!

Selecting an Exercise Program

How do you as a diabetic select an exercise program for yourself? Exactly the same way anyone else does! Determine what sports in which you like to participate. No one else can choose for you. To work out regularly, you must pick a group of activities you will enjoy. It is pointless to take up jogging if you dislike the activity. You will not stick with it, and whatever you do choose must become a part of your routine forever, or until you can replace it with another activity of equal effort.

In the following pages you'll find many activity choices. Each type of exercise has a specific benefit. It is up to you to put together several of these exercises, the sum total of which will be your own workout program. Keep in mind the following points as you make up your own program:

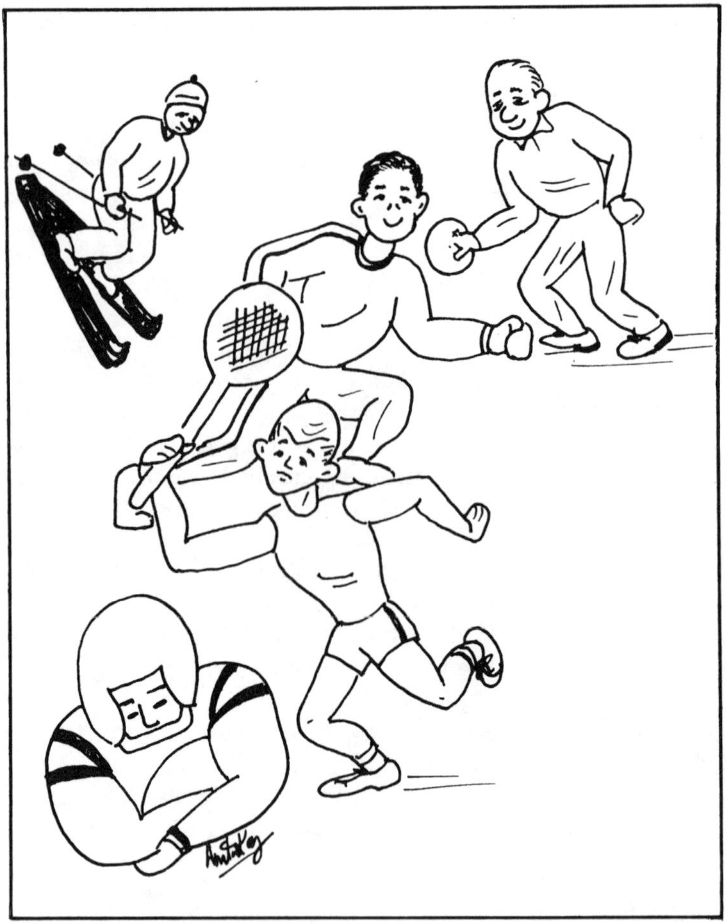

Fig. 2-11. Regular daily exercise is important for proper control of diabetes.

• What areas of your body do you want to improve? If you want to develop stamina, improve your cardiovascular system, and flatten your stomach muscles, you will develop a different program than the person who wants to slim her legs and fanny and build up her bust. Both are legitimate goals, but vastly different programs will be needed.

• What do you enjoy? A tremendous variety of exercises is available to you. Pick a program with which you can have fun. Don't let someone else pick a program for you and expect to enjoy it as much as one you select yourself.

• What is convenient to you? Unless you live on the east coast of England, don't pick channel swimming as your game. If you love to swim, you'll have better luck finding a lap pool. Do not pick events that are hard to get to. It's great to do five miles of cross-country skiing daily. There is no better exercise, but if you must drive 50 miles every day to get to the snow, your enthusiasm won't last. Inconvenience is one of the greatest causes of attrition. Don't make it tough on yourself.

- What can you do with others? Whenever possible, try to get someone you really like involved with you (Fig. 2-12). If you can tolerate racquetball, and your best friend loves it, pick racquetball as one of your activities. His enthusiasm will keep you both going. It is best if you are both at about the same level of play. If he is an expert and you're a duffer, it won't work for either of you. Anything you can do with your spouse or family is an excellent choice. Studies

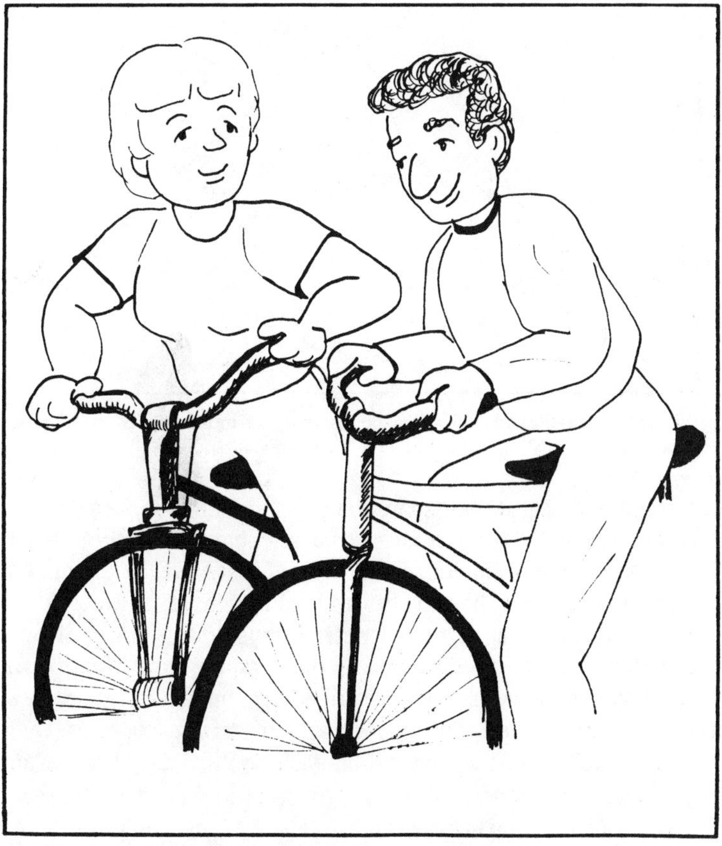

Fig. 2-12. Find a partner for your exercise program.

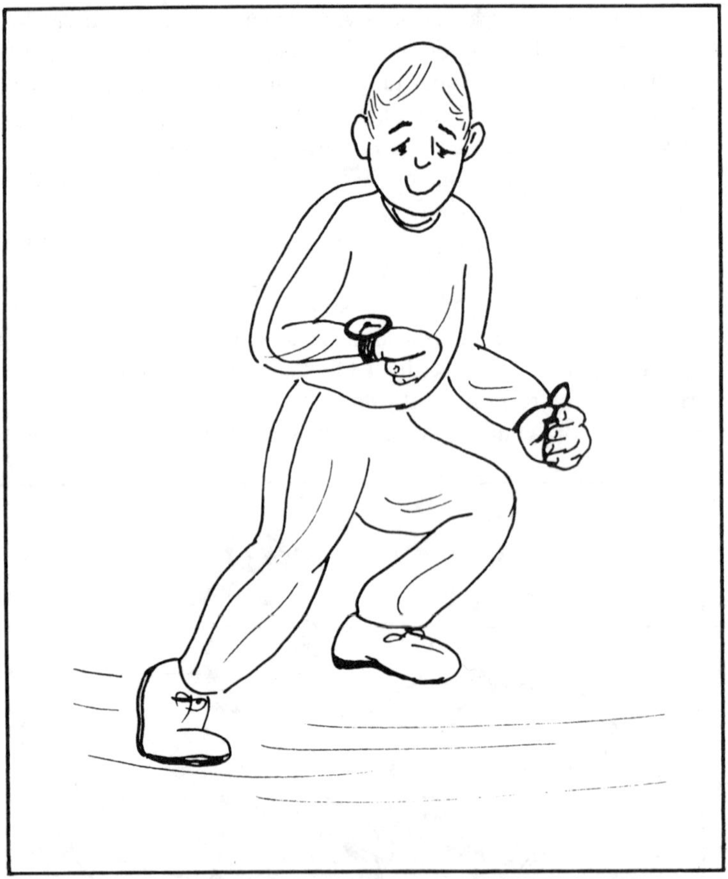

Fig. 2-13. Walking is an ideal exercise and the most natural to humans. It requires no special training and little if any special equipment.

have shown that if your spouse supports you in your program, you have over an 80 percent chance for sticking with it (Fig. 2-14).

• What will challenge you? When I first started walking, I was bored to death. I walked my first mile in 19 minutes and felt it did me no good. The second mile I pushed myself and did in about 16 minutes. It made my heart pump quite rapidly, my breath burn a little, and my legs ache. It was still boring, but at least it seemed to be doing some good. The indoor track I walk is 16 laps to the mile. I found out that if I time myself on each lap, it is less boring, and I could have better control over my overall time. I figured out that if I could walk each lap in 56 seconds, I'd be walking 4 miles an hour, or a 15-minute mile. That gave me a personal challenge and relieved a lot of the boredom. It wasn't long before I could walk a routine 15-minute mile without too much discomfort; so I set my goal at a 14-minute mile or a 52-second lap. Taking 4 seconds off of each lap didn't sound like much, and it wasn't difficult to keep up that pace for a couple of laps. By the end of the second week I did a 13:50 mile.

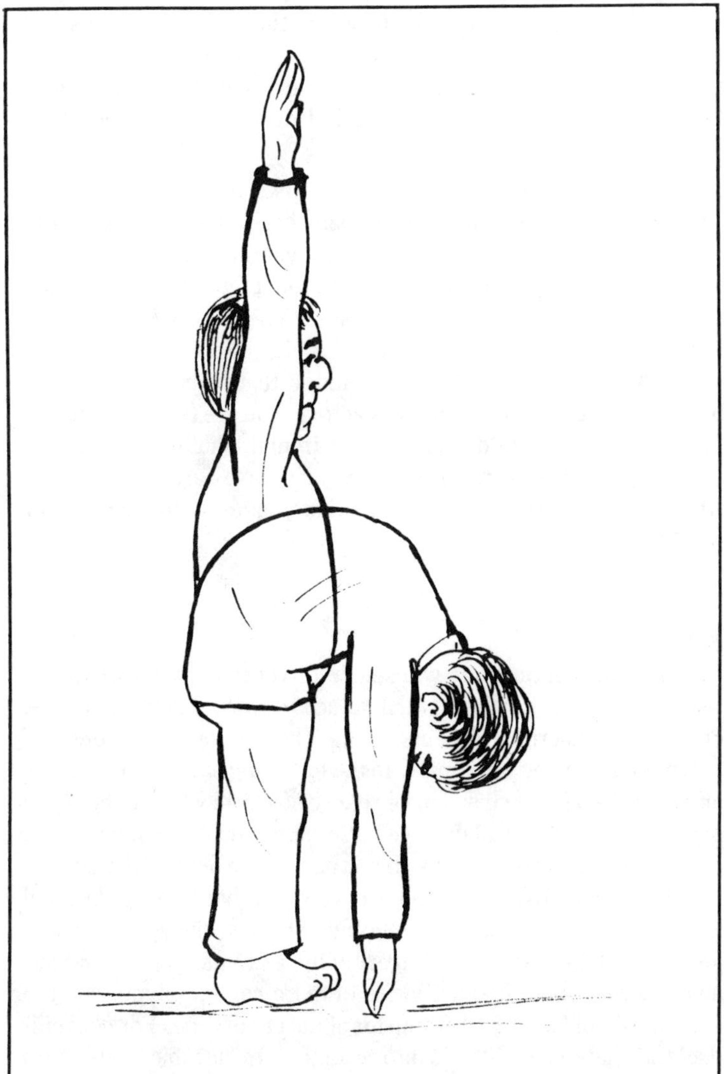

Fig. 2-14. Warm-up exercises can prevent injury and fill in on rare days when you can't get to your regular program.

My next challenge was a 13:30 mile, or a lap every 49:5 seconds. That took another week. Now I'm shooting for a 12-minute mile, or 16 laps at 45 seconds each. It will take me a while to get there, but it keeps me going at a task I originally found boring. I try to walk my daily miles in about 14 minutes routinely and a record mile only once a week.

Challenging yourself with distances, times, or repetitions will keep you interested in your workouts. The best part of a challenge is that making it becomes a powerful reward in itself. Don't set your challenges unrealistically. Leave the 4-minute mile to the other guy.

• Along with the exercises you choose for yourself, there are a few things you should include on a daily basis. These are warm-up exercises to ensure that you won't injure your muscles. Also, these exercises will keep you from losing ground if there are times when you just have to miss a complete workout. They can be done in a few minutes almost anywhere (Fig. 2-15).

• Another thing to keep in mind is that if the program you choose doesn't turn out to be satisfactory, you are free to change it in any way you like. Add to it, subtract from it, shuffle it around, do different programs on different days; just make sure you do some form of vigorous exercise everyday that you aren't too sick to get out of bed.

Your Workout Program

The workout program you select for yourself should be determined largely by what you want to accomplish. There should be aerobic and anaerobic aspects to it. The proportions should be determined again by your goals. In the following pages I will discuss a number of aerobic and anaerobic exercises from which to help you choose. To list all available exercise activities is far beyond the scope of this or any other book. If you have some pet activity such as log rolling, don't expect to find it covered in these pages, but feel free to do your log rolling. Any activity which works your muscles, heart, and lungs without endangering life and limb is good and fair game. Herein you'll find activities of more common type, and the selection should offer something for almost everyone. For convenience, they have been divided into aerobic and anaerobic types, with a discussion of advantages and disadvantages for each.

Aerobic Exercises. *Aerobic exercises* are those which utilize maximum oxygen. They work the heart and lungs for longer periods

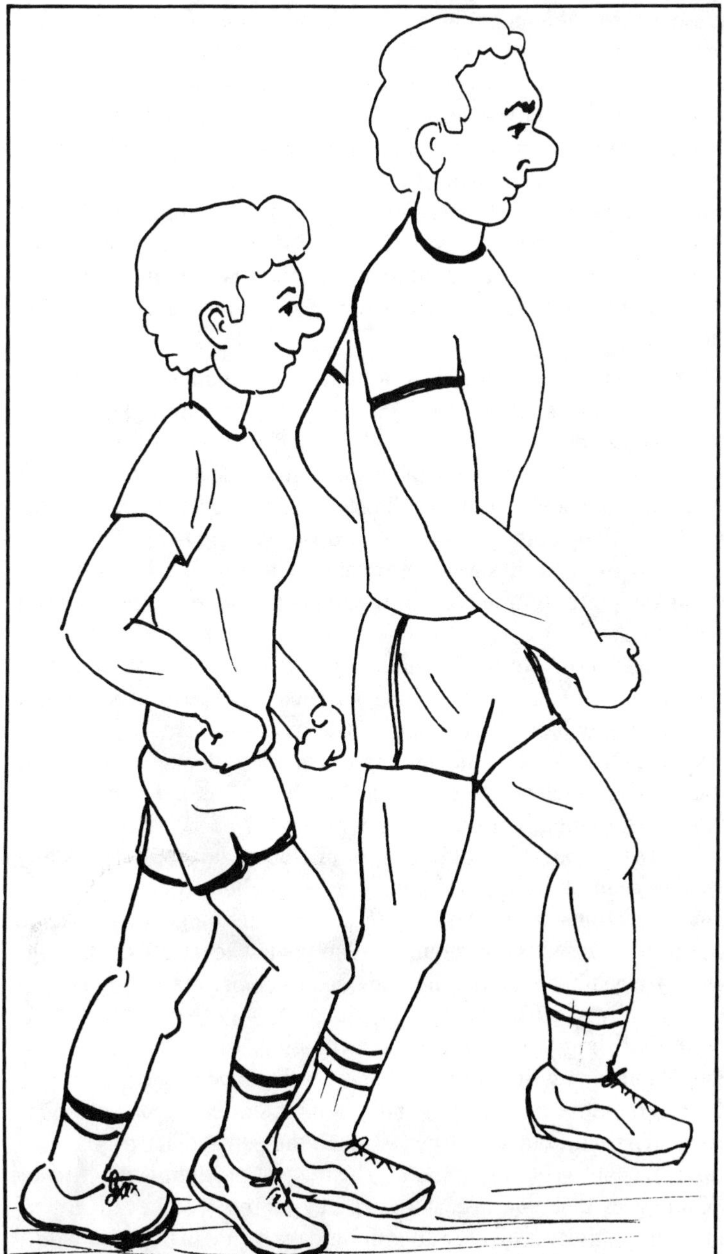

Fig. 2-15. A brisk walk can be taken at almost anytime and any place. It is one of the best aerobic workouts if pursued for even half an hour.

at a time than the anaerobics. This does not mean that anaerobics don't burn oxygen or speed the heart. All activity does, but anaerobics usually work muscles against resistance for short spurts of time and do not exercise the heart and lungs sufficiently. Aerobics tend to increase endurance while toning and building muscles. The total amount of work you perform during aerobics is usually cumulatively greater; so you usually burn more calories and storage fat, since they are generally carried out for longer periods of time. It has been estimated that the first two minutes of any exercise are anaerobic, utilizing energy stored within the muscles themselves.

- Walking—A brisk walk for one or two miles or more is excellent exercise (Figs. 2-13 through 2-15). It requires no equipment and can be done almost anywhere and anytime. It is beneficial to get a special pair of comfortable shoes and to do it where there is a minimum of traffic. It is the most natural exercise available to mankind. Many authorities feel that brisk walking is even superior to jogging in that it has less potential for injuring your back or knee and ankle joints. A mile done in 16 minutes or faster is considered a brisk walk.
- Jogging—Like brisk walking, jogging is an aerobic exercise that can be done almost anywhere, anytime (Fig. 2-16). It requires a minimum of equipment, though a little more than walking. A good pair of running shoes and running clothes are almost essential. If you have a tendency toward back problems or knee and ankle weaknesses, jogging may not be for you.
- Swimming—Though swimming does not burn as many calories as brisk walking or jogging, it is excellent because it works many more muscles of the body (Fig. 2-17). Its biggest handicap is that to do it effectively requires a lap pool at least 25 yards long. They are readily available in many health clubs, but you must join such a facility to use them.
- Bicycling—Bicycling, like swimming, utilizes many of the body's muscles with more emphasis on the lower limbs. It can be done outside on a vehicle or indoors on a stationary bicycle (Fig. 2-18). The workout you'll get is much the same. There is a wide range of cost to such equipment. The biggest problem with outdoor bicycling is that you are at the mercy of the weather. Have an alternate activity available to you on days you can't get outside.
- Rope skipping—Rope skipping is an excellent aerobic exercise (Fig. 2-19). It requires some skill, but it can be mastered by most of us. It takes a minimum of space and equipment and is not

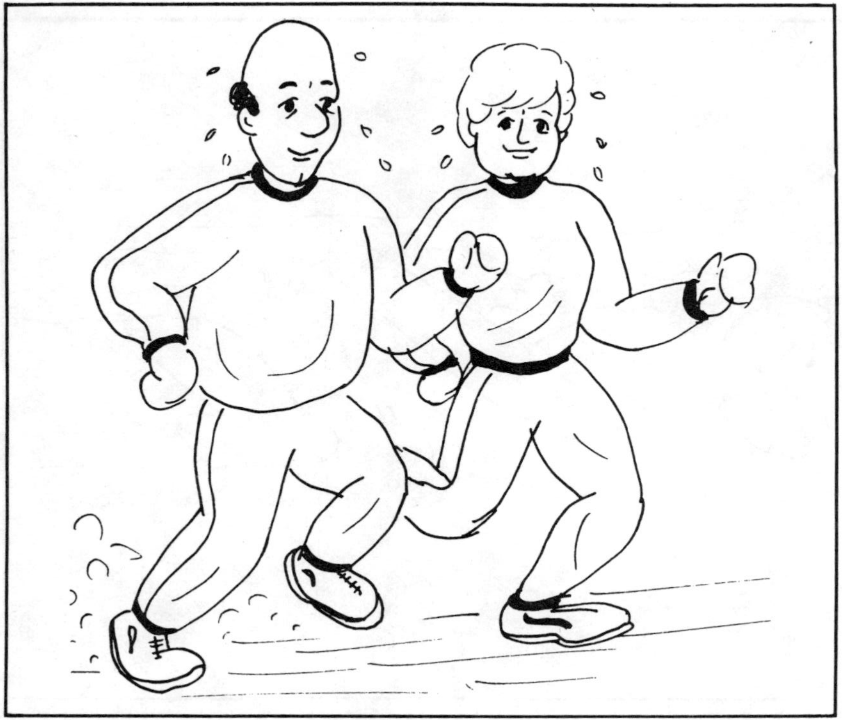

Fig. 2-16. Jogging is also an excellent aerobic workout but more traumatic to joints and backs than walking.

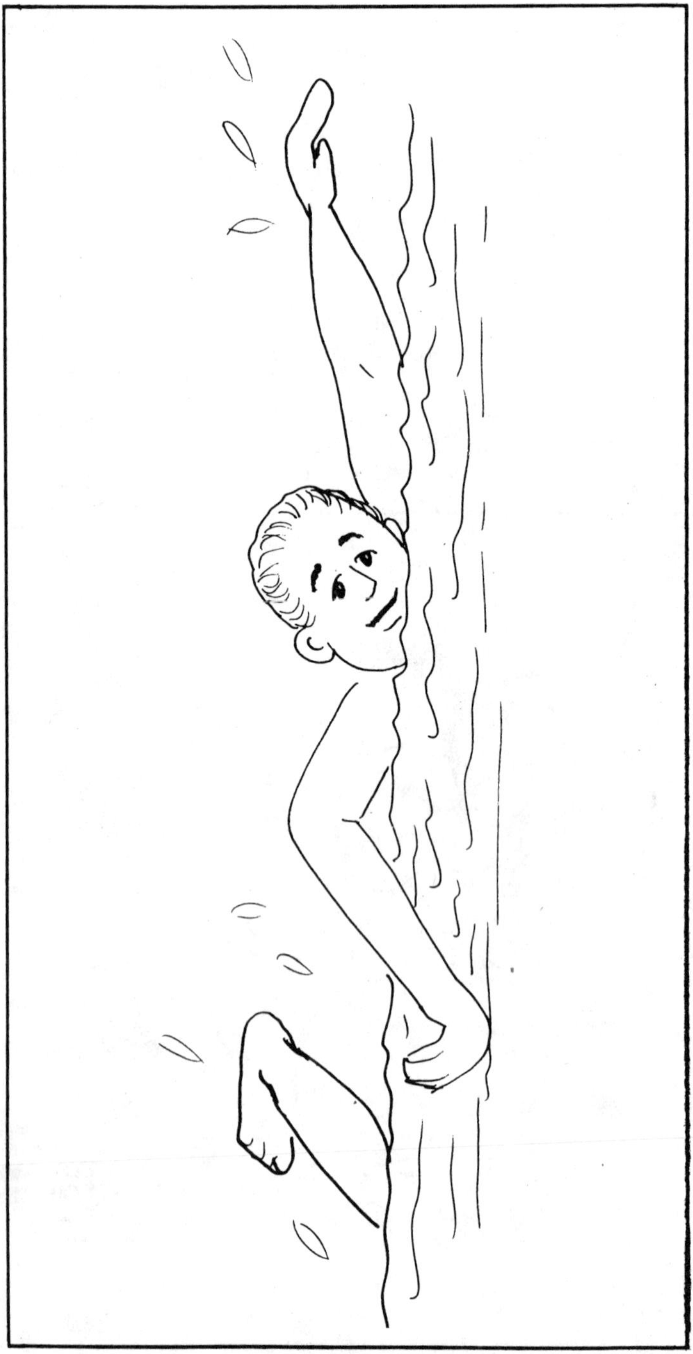

Fig. 2-17. Swimming works almost all muscles of the body.

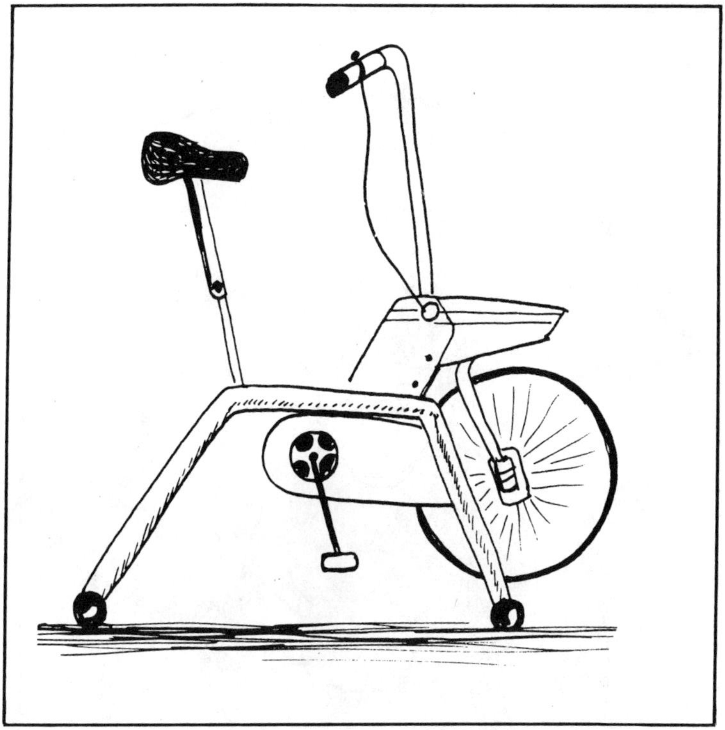

Fig. 2-18. Bicycle riding is a great exercise both indoors and out.

subject to weather changes. Consider it in combination with other activities you enjoy.

• Racquetball—Racquetball is an easy sport to learn. If played vigorously, it gives you a terrific workout. You just about have to join a club to play this game, and of course you need a partner (Fig. 2-20). Equipment has a wide range of cost but need not be expensive. Since it is an indoor sport, weather does not affect it.

• Tennis—Unless you are a very good tennis player and keep constantly moving, you may not be getting the workout you want (Fig. 2-21). The way some people play this game could almost be considered anaerobic. It takes long volleys to really get a good workout in tennis. Long volleys usually require good players.

• Team sports—The biggest problem with team sports is that usually they are seasonal, and games and practices may not be daily. Unless it's a game like basketball, soccer, or volleyball, you may not move much (Fig. 2-22). In football and baseball, you may stand around waiting for plays for such long periods that you get virtually

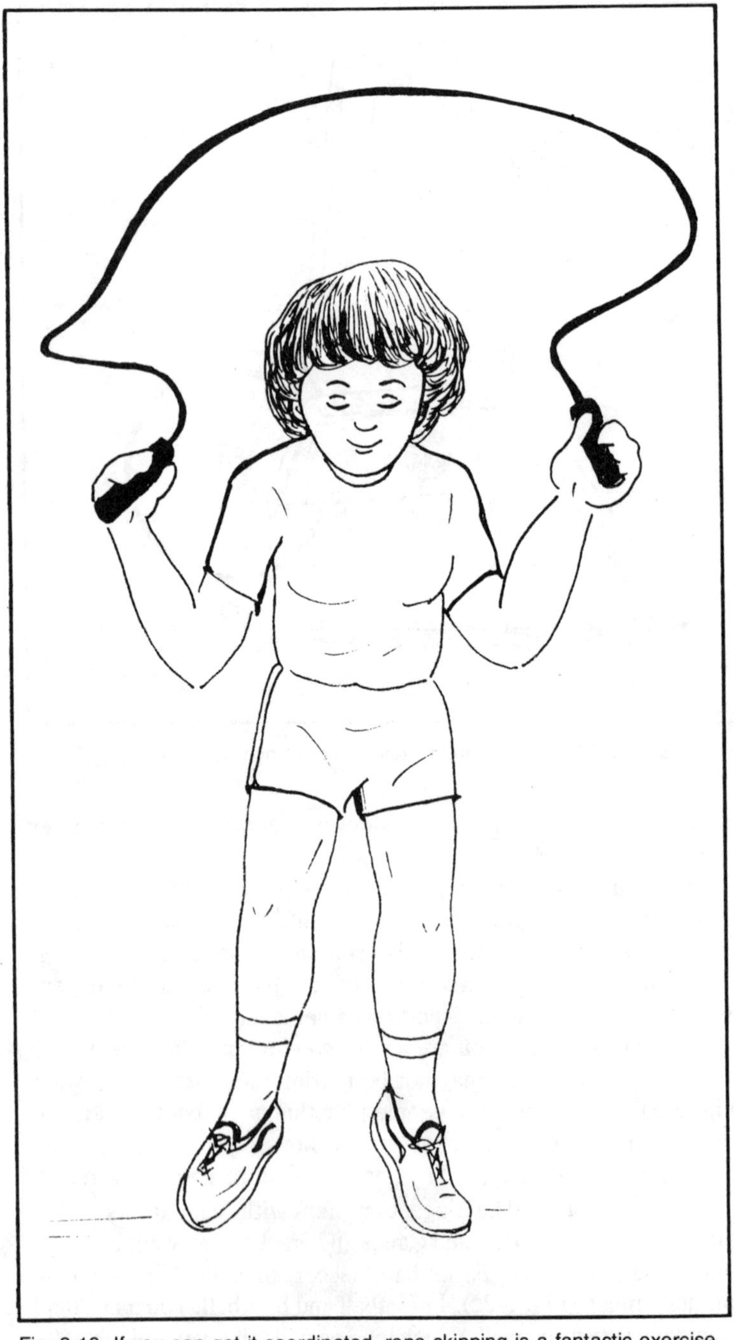

Fig. 2-19. If you can get it coordinated, rope skipping is a fantastic exercise.

no workout. Because of the short spurts of running and activity, football and baseball must be considered anaerobic.

• Golf—If you walk quickly and carry your own clubs, golf can be a good game (Fig. 2-23). But for most of us, our game works out the caddy or runs up the mileage on the golf cart. It is also a relatively expensive game, and too few of us can do it on a daily basis.

• Aerobic dancing and exercises—Jazzercise and aerobic dancing and exercise classes have taken the country by storm, and it's a good storm (Fig. 2-24). A well supervised program gives you an excellent and fun workout if you like this type of thing. There are even excellent video programs that you can use at home. Equipment is usually limited to workout clothes and shoes, which need not be expensive. There is a fairly wide range of costs for the classes, but if you shop around you can find them for around 5 dollars a session or less.

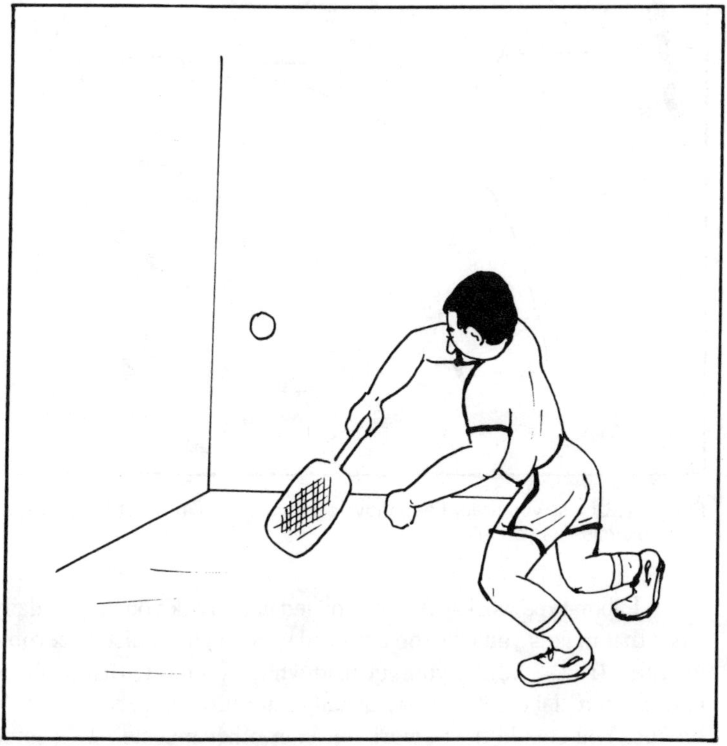

Fig. 2-20. Racquet ball requires a partner, and you'll probably have to join a club, but it is a terrific workout and challenge.

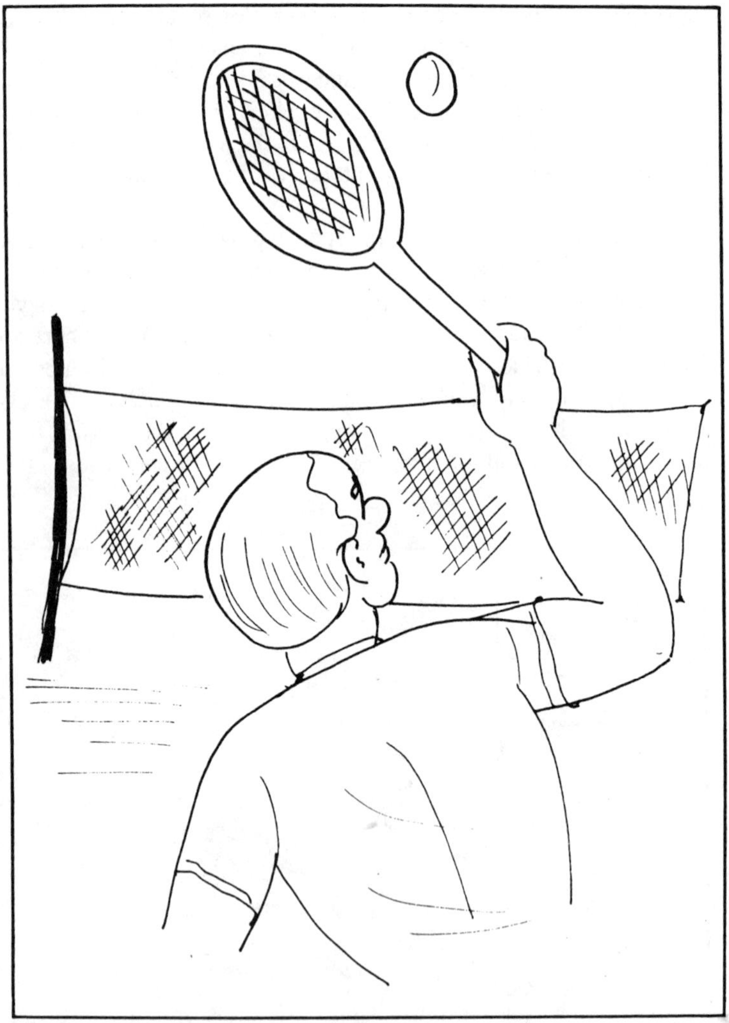

Fig. 2-21. Unless you really keep moving in tennis, you may not be getting as much exercise as you think.

• Labor-type work—Any prolonged hard work you do on a daily basis that makes you breathe hard and speeds your pulse is aerobic exercise (Fig. 2-25). If you get paid while you do it, that's all the better. Hard labor, however, usually only utilizes certain muscle groups. You should try to work out your other muscles with some additional exercises.

• Once in a while and team sports—Skiing, skating, basketball,

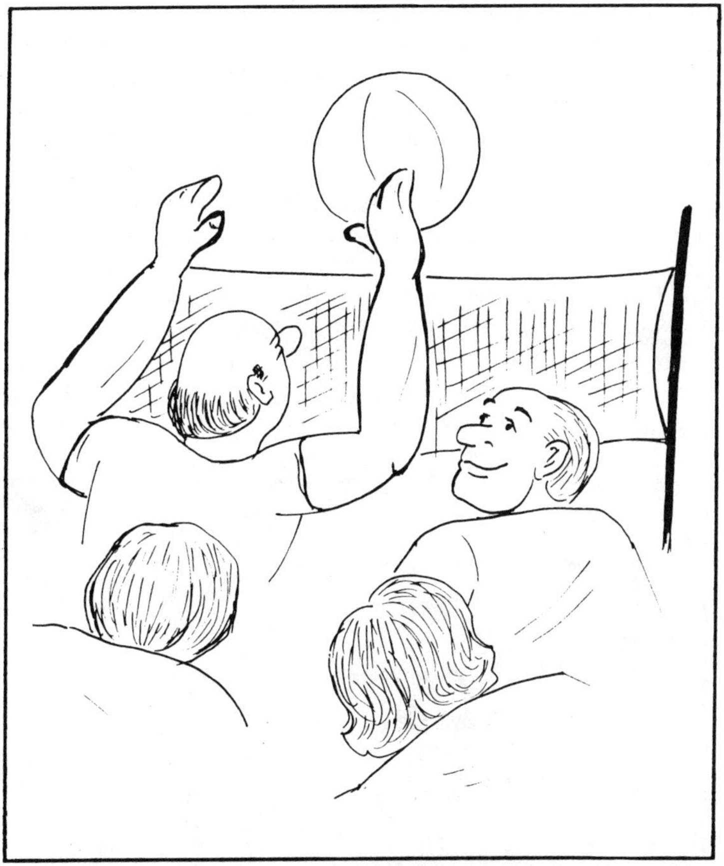

Fig. 2-22. Team sports are fine if you participate often enough and regularly.

and volleyball are all excellent aerobic exercises. Unless they are done on a regular and frequent basis, however, they will not satisfy your needs. If you are involved in these type of activities, make sure you do some other equally vigorous workout on alternate days (Fig. 2-26).

Anaerobics. *Anaerobic exercises* are those which utilize muscular activity for short spurts of time. They do little for your cardiovascular system, although they may strengthen you tremendously. It is important that you mix aerobic exercises with your anaerobic program if body building and strength training are important to you. Anaerobics are important to those who want to gain weight or sculpture their physique in a particular way.

- Weight lifting—There are two types of weight-training programs. One is to develop enormous strength to compete in weight-lifting competition. The people who engage in this type of training are power lifters and work with heavy weights. The second type of weight training is for the individual who wants to sculpture a "body beautiful." This person usually works with less weight, but he repeats the specific exercises designed to work on individual muscle groups many times. The latter may almost get into the area of aerobics. If you are interested in this type of workout, get some good coaching (Fig. 2-27).

• Exercises and everyday activity—Many exercises can only be kept up for short periods of time, such as push-ups, sit-ups, chinning, etc. (Fig. 2-28), so they are anaerobic. The same goes for many of the activities we do daily; climbing stairs, walking short distances, lifting groceries and other loads, etc. They keep certain

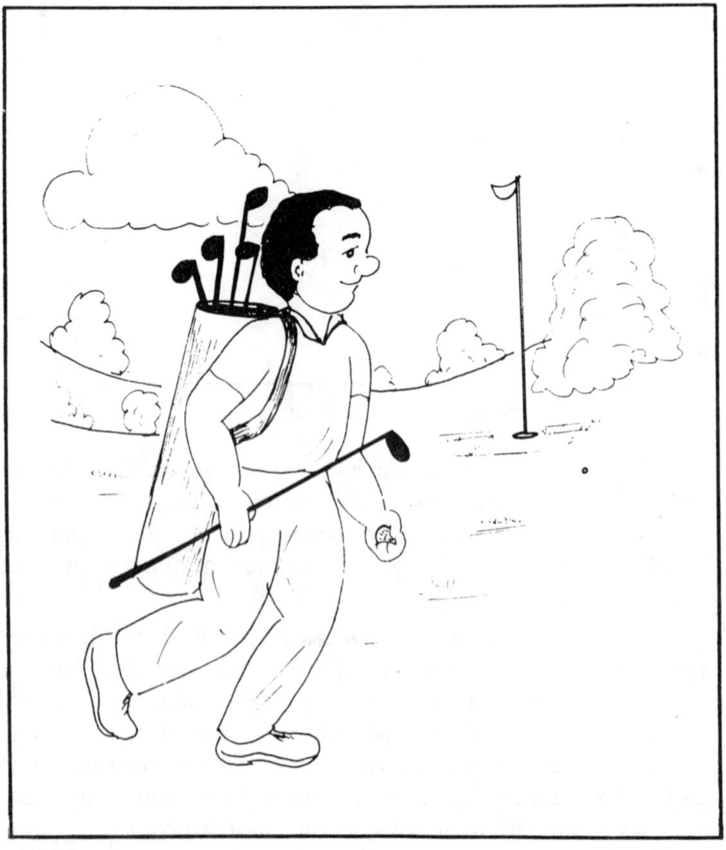

Fig. 2-23. If golf is your game, walk—don't let the caddy and cart do all the work.

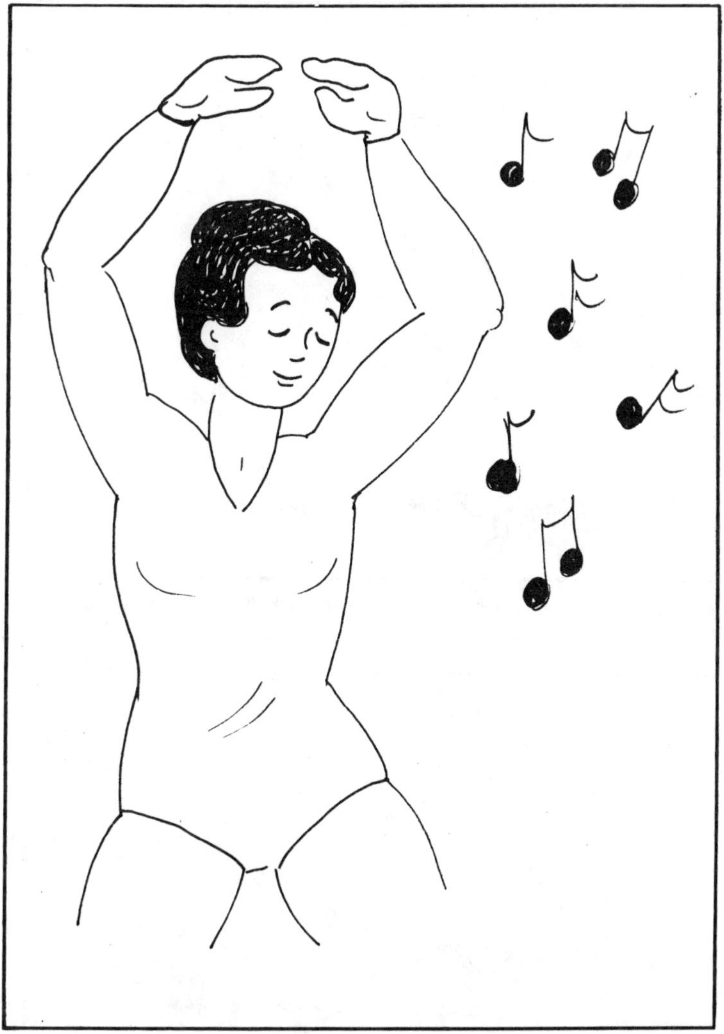

Fig. 2-24. Aerobic classes are fantastic not only for exercise but to make new contacts and friends.

of our muscles active and in tone if our occupations make us do them all the time, but they do little for our general fitness. You may end up as the patient with the biggest bicep in the cardiac ward if you don't work out the rest of your body and cardiovascular system. You can get great benefit from everyday activities though, if you make the effort. Always walk stairs instead of taking elevators. Don't pick the parking place nearest the door of the place to which you're

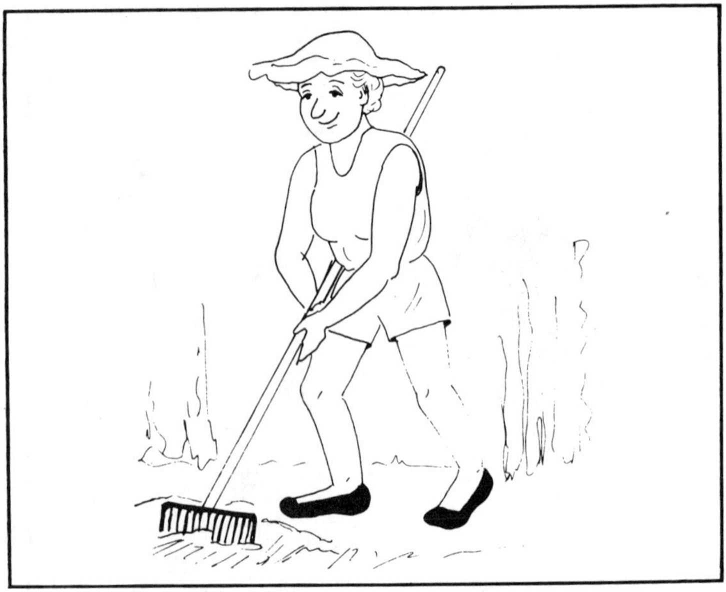

Fig. 2-25. Labor is good if it is daily and makes you huff and puff for a prolonged period.

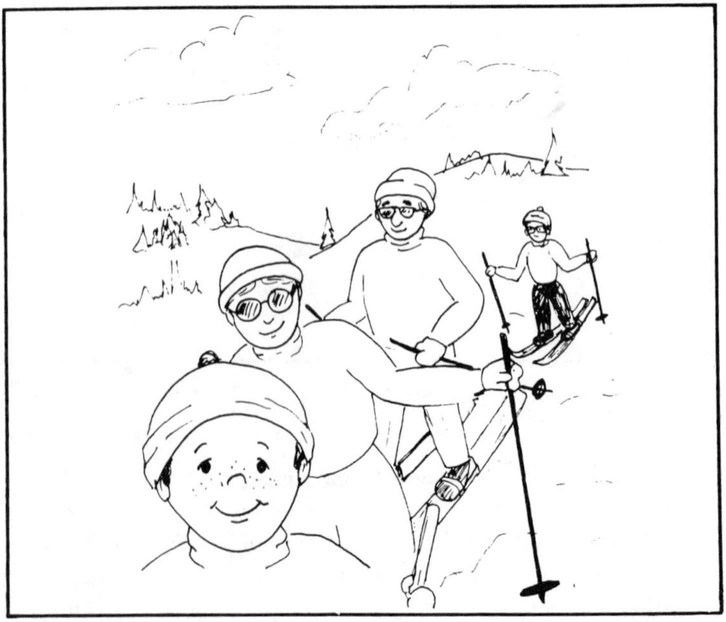

Fig. 2-26. The problem with some of the best exercises is that they cannot be done on a regular enough basis. Exercise must be done daily.

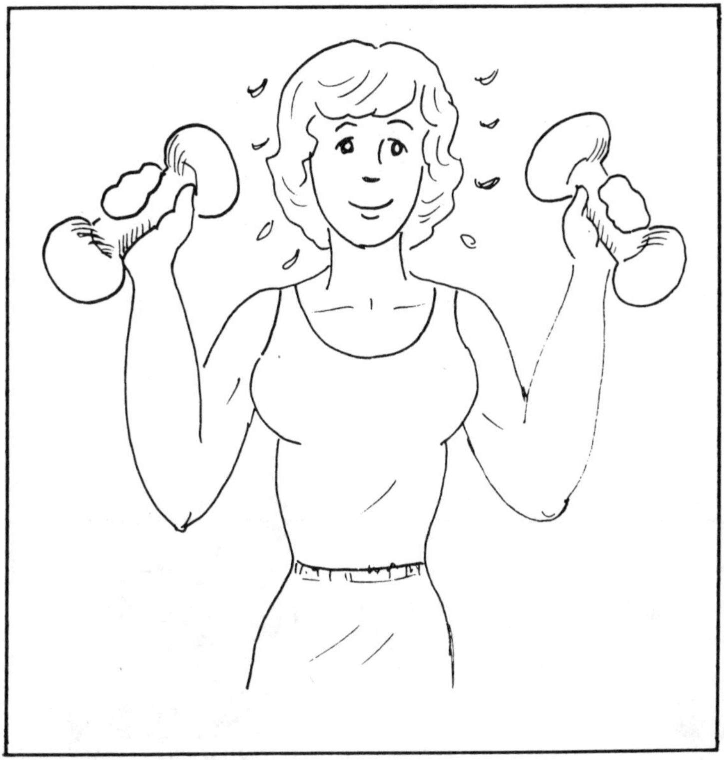

Fig. 2-27. Weight lifting has become very popular among both men and women. It is essential that you get good coaching for the best benefit and avoidance of injury.

going. When you have only a few blocks to go, don't drive, walk briskly. Don't always ask others to do heavy work for you. To be effective these activities must be done regularly and daily.

• Once in a while and team sports—Like those team sports mentioned under aerobics, anaerobic team sports must be participated in frequently and regularly to do any good (Fig. 2-29). It surprises many people to find out that football and baseball are usually considered anaerobic sports, as is bowling. Any sport that involves short spurts of activity—less than 2 minutes of continuous work—are usually considered anaerobic. They tend to require more skill than endurance.

SUMMARY

Exercise on a regular daily schedule is important to anyone,

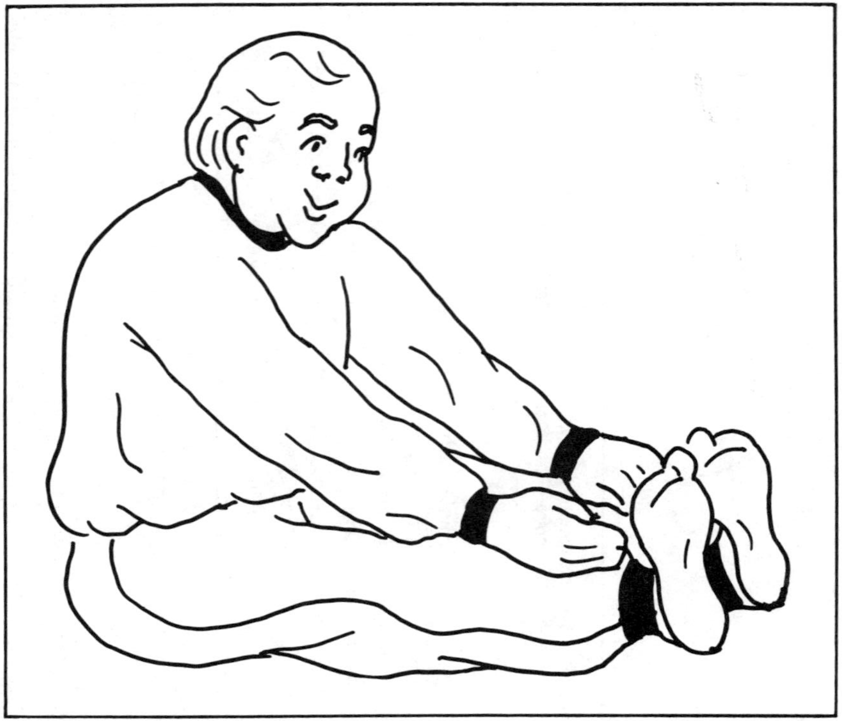

Fig. 2-28. Many exercises can be done in the home with little or no expense.

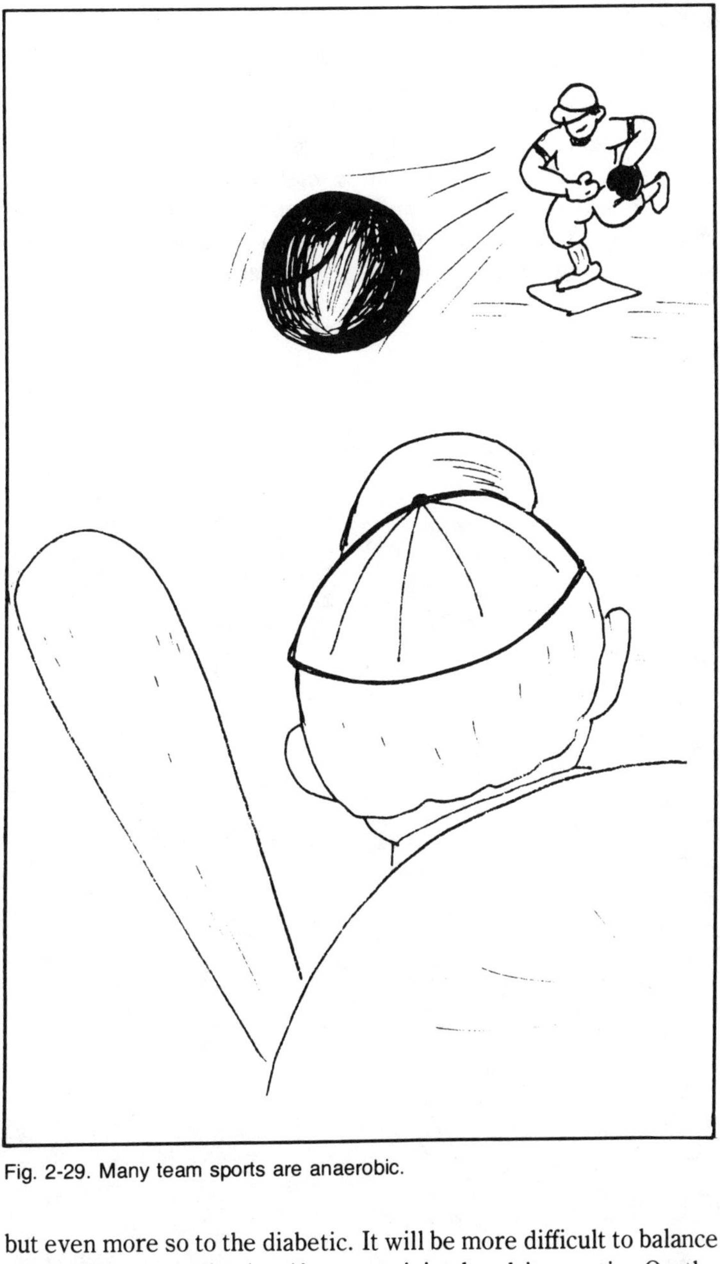

Fig. 2-29. Many team sports are anaerobic.

but even more so to the diabetic. It will be more difficult to balance your diet and medication if your activity level is erratic. On the other hand, if you maintain a high activity level, balancing will be much easier. Go over your daily activities, work, and exercise very precisely with your physician. If there are days when you are less active, for example, weekends, he may want to adjust your medication or diet on those days. Consistency is of greater importance to the diabetic than the nondiabetic.

Hopefully, this chapter has given you some insight into the importance and roles of medication, diet, and activity in your daily life. When your physician works with you to evaluate and prescribe your regimen, discuss it with him. Your intelligent input is important in coming up with a successful program.

3: Living a Normal Life with Your Diabetes

IN THE BEGINNING OF THIS BOOK, WE SAW A COMMON quote among diabetics, "Diabetes is the best incurable disease someone could have!" They feel this way because they are able to live perfectly normal lives, pursuing whatever goals they've set for themselves. Their lives are full, rewarding, and happy. Yet there are some who feel that because they are diabetic, life has dealt them a terrible hand. Consciously or subconsciously they feel inferior, that diabetes is something to be ashamed of, that they are less than whole. They rebel against their diet, their medication, and often their physician and loved ones who are trying to help them. Their poor state of mind and poor self-esteem are their worst enemies. In some cases professional psychiatric help may be necessary before they can get on with their lives. Fortunately, these cases are rare, a very small percentage of all diabetics. If the problem is recognized, however, it should not be taken lightly. Help should be sought immediately.

SUPPORT GROUPS

Some, but sadly not enough, areas have diabetes support groups (Fig. 3-1). They are a boon to new diabetics and helpful to long timers as well. Check with your physician, local hospital, nearest National Diabetic Association office, social workers, or local health department for information regarding a diabetes support group in your area.

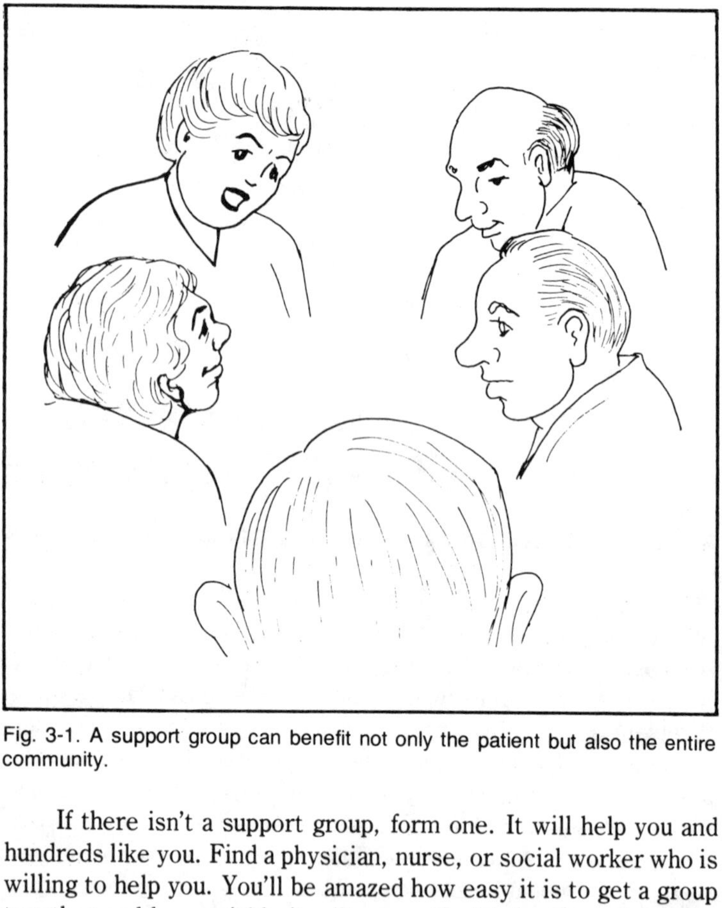

Fig. 3-1. A support group can benefit not only the patient but also the entire community.

If there isn't a support group, form one. It will help you and hundreds like you. Find a physician, nurse, or social worker who is willing to help you. You'll be amazed how easy it is to get a group together and how quickly it will grow. You'll also be delighted at how much you benefit by it. Your physician or local hospital will be able to put you in touch with many other diabetics who are interested in helping you get a support group together.

What is the purpose of a diabetic support group? Basically it is to offer help to diabetics and their families. The following is a list of just a few of the services a diabetes support group can offer its members and its community. It can:

• Disseminate information about diabetes to the community. They can make the general public understand the disease and dispel myths about diabetes and diabetics.

• Campaign to get the general public to get checked for diabetes. Early diagnosis is important for prevention of secondary health problems caused by diabetes, such as heart disease, stroke, renal disease, hardening of the arteries, hypertension, neurological problems, and visual problems.

• Help newly diagnosed diabetics and their familes to understand and cope with their diseases. They can give them a place to call for information and help, as well as help them belong.

• Keep up with new developments in the research of the disease, its treatment, and dynamics. Members have a place to share information they've acquired with others. Lectures can be sponsored for the membership and community.

• Provide a social group for people with a common interest and problem. This is not to say that diabetics don't fit into all social groups. They do, but often we develop new friends and special fondness among people who share special problems with us.

• Provide a lobby. It is more effective when a large group of people speak with one voice to get merchants, schools, or the community to become sensitive to special needs of the group members.

LIVING A FULL LIFE

All your goals and efforts as a diabetic should be aimed at making your life as near to what it would have been if you weren't a diabetic. In all but a very few cases, there should be no limits on your horizon. Diabetics have been successful in all walks of life—sports, business, stage, screen, television, radio, politics, clergy, law, medicine, even in the military. There is no goal that you can't set for yourself as a diabetic!

If your physician cannot work with you to get your diabetes under control so that you can get on with a normal life, then it is time to get a second opinion. It is a rare diabetic who can't get his or her life back on track, but the diabetic must cooperate and work at it. The few sacrifices and small added effort are worth the tremendous reward of a fruitful future.

Monitoring Blood Sugar

To live a full and normal life as a diabetic means keeping your blood sugar in a normal range. There are several ways to monitor your blood sugar. One way is to go to your physician's office or a hospital lab and get frequent blood sugars drawn and urines tested. This is expensive and inconvenient. Once you are under reasonable control, your physician should "wean" you to be able to test yourself, turning much of the responsibility of maintaining your balance over to you, where it really belongs (Figs. 3-2 and 3-3). There are numerous methods for the diabetic to assess his or her control:

Urine Tests. Tes-Tape is a paper tape that measures the presence of sugar in your urine. It is a simple test which requires dipping a small strip of the tape in your urine sample—a few drops will do—and watching for color changes on the tape. The Tes-Tape will remain yellow if there is no sugar spilling over in your urine, meaning that your blood sugar is below elevated levels. If your blood sugar is elevated it should spill over into your urine, and the Tes-Tape will turn green or blue within 60 seconds. Testing your urine three or four times a day will tell you how to adjust your medication, diet, or exercise according to a program outlined for you by your physician. Testing your urine three or four times a day will tell you how to adjust your medication, diet, or exercise according to a program outlined for you by your physician.

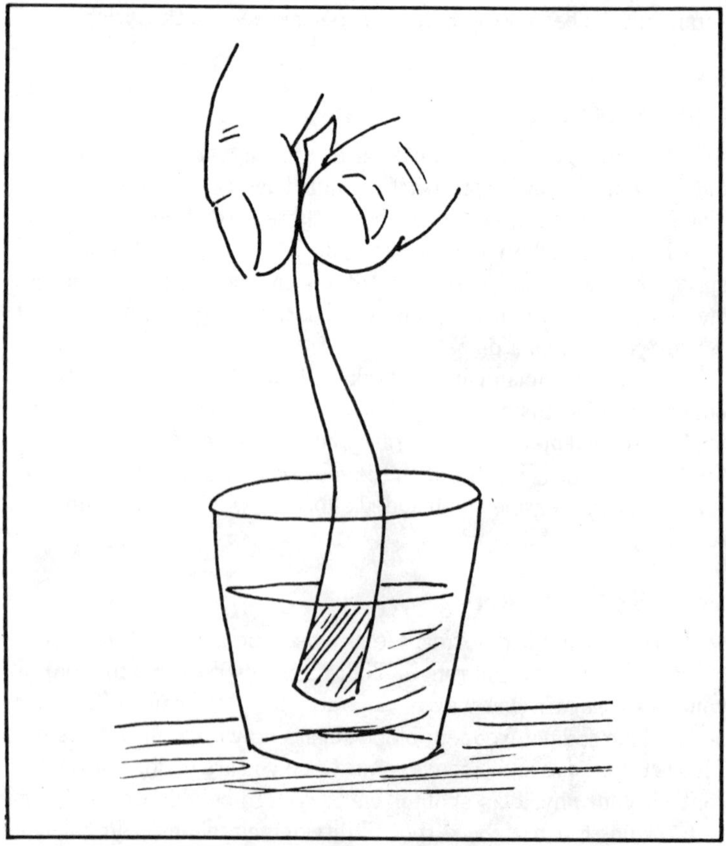

Fig. 3-2. It is a simple matter to test your own urine sugar.

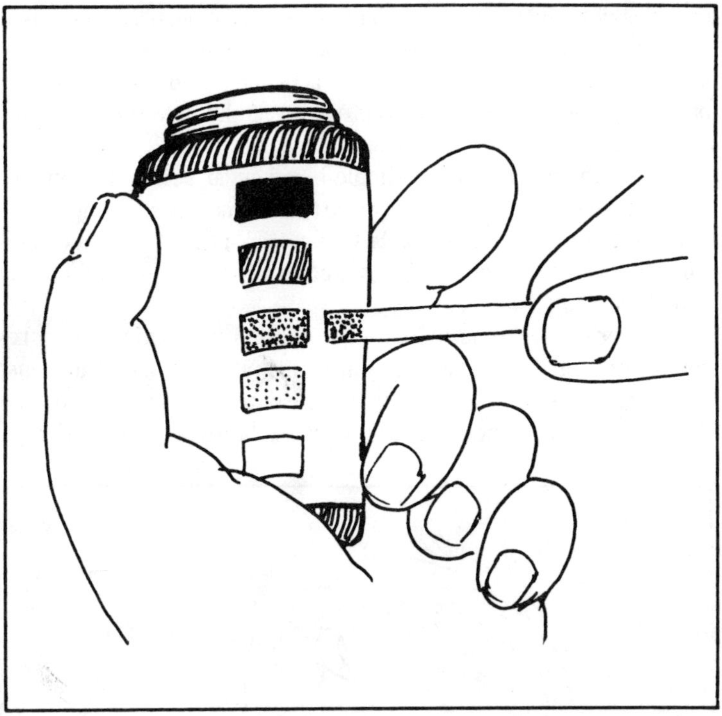

Fig. 3-3. There are a number of brands and methods for self-testing, each with its own advantages. Select your method with your doctor. Some tests are more sensitive than others. Your needs should determine which is best for you.

Diastix is a similar method to measure sugar spilling in your urine. Its advantage over Tes-Tape is a more accurate quantitative measure of how much sugar is spilling, making it easier for your physician to fine-tune your program of diet, activity, and medication. The Diastix has a greater array of color changes which can be compared to a chart on the bottle, thus giving a more specific reading of sugar levels.

Clinitest is a more cumbersome chemical color test, but even more accurate and specific than either test tape or dip-stick methods (Fig. 3-4). Most diabetics do not need this degree of accuracy. For the occasional diabetic who is having a difficult time adjusting his or her program, the rare *brittle diabetic*, the Clinitest is a valuable measure.

Blood Sugar Tests. Until recent years diabetics had to go to their physician's office or to a medical lab to have a blood sugar evaluated. New technology has made self-testing of blood sugar now possible. This capability has many advantages. Not only is it cheaper and more convenient to be able to self test your blood sugar, it also gives the physician a practical method of checking on a patient's blood sugar at various times of the day under normal activities.

The Chemstrip bG is a simple blood sugar self-testing kit not unlike the test tape or dip-stick urine testing methods. A single drop of blood obtained from a simple finger stick is applied to a chemically treated strip, which changes color to indicate quantitatively your blood sugar level.

Several electronic blood sugar self-testing devices have recently come on the market. They are still quite expensive, and most diabetics do not need them. For that small percentage who do need them to fine tune their diabetic control, however, they offer far

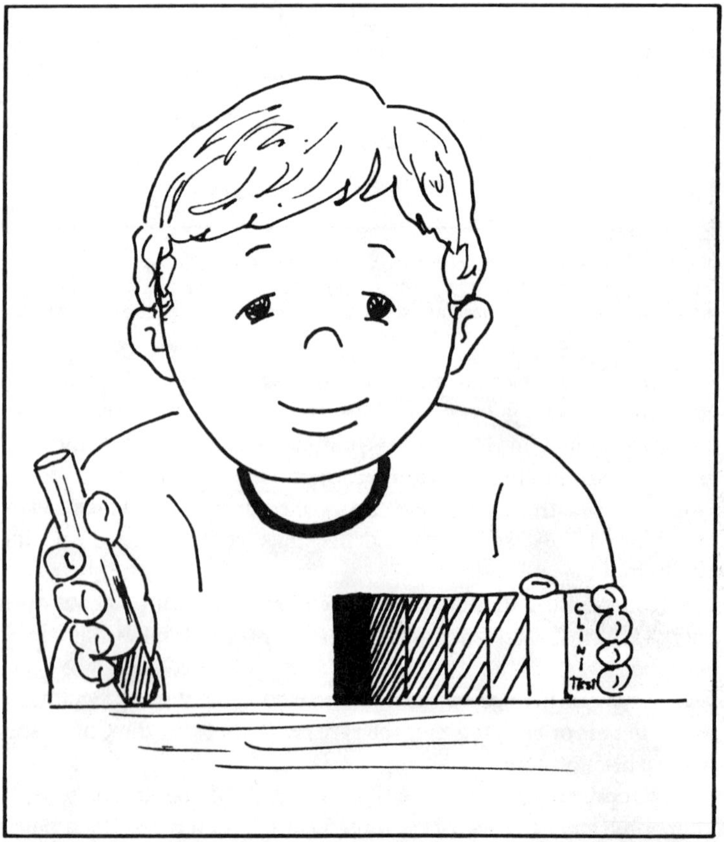

Fig. 3-4. For the "brittle diabetic," the Clinitest is a valuable measure.

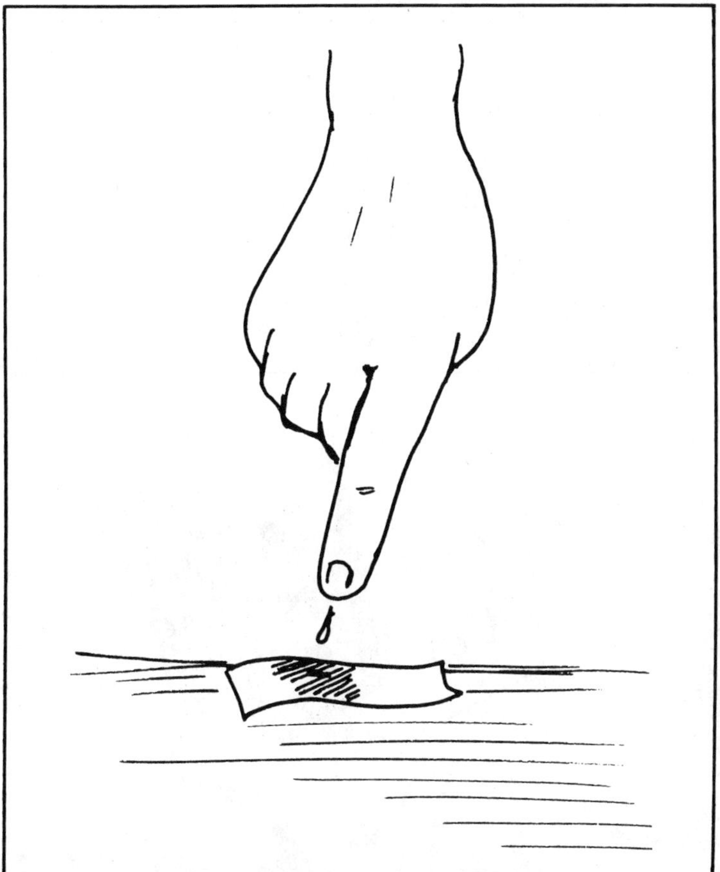

Fig. 3-5. Blood sugar can also be tested by simple methods.

greater accuracy than the chemical method. Most of these devices work on batteries and are portable.

These self-testing devices are a boon to physician and patient in trying to achieve good diabetic control (Figs. 3-5 and 3-6). Careful use and recording of results will give your doctor the information he needs to help you to a course of good health and normal activity.

Enjoying Activities

Once you and your physician have worked out a program that works for you, you should be able to enjoy most of the activities you've always enjoyed. Eating out, for example, should not be a

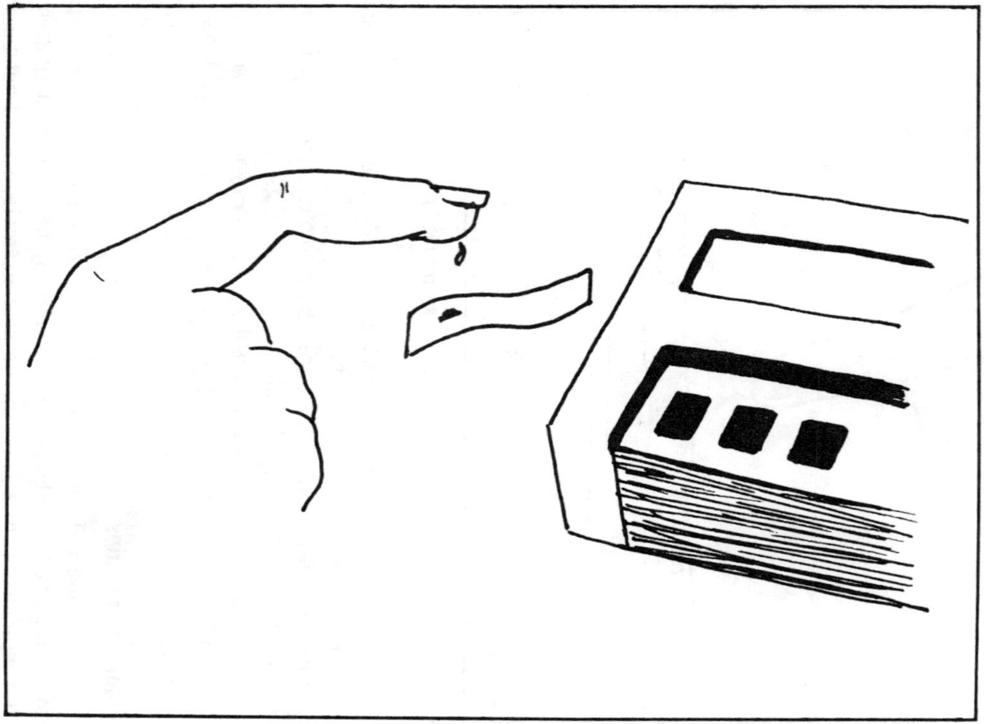

Fig. 3-6. New electronic self-testing devices are now available to the diabetic patient.

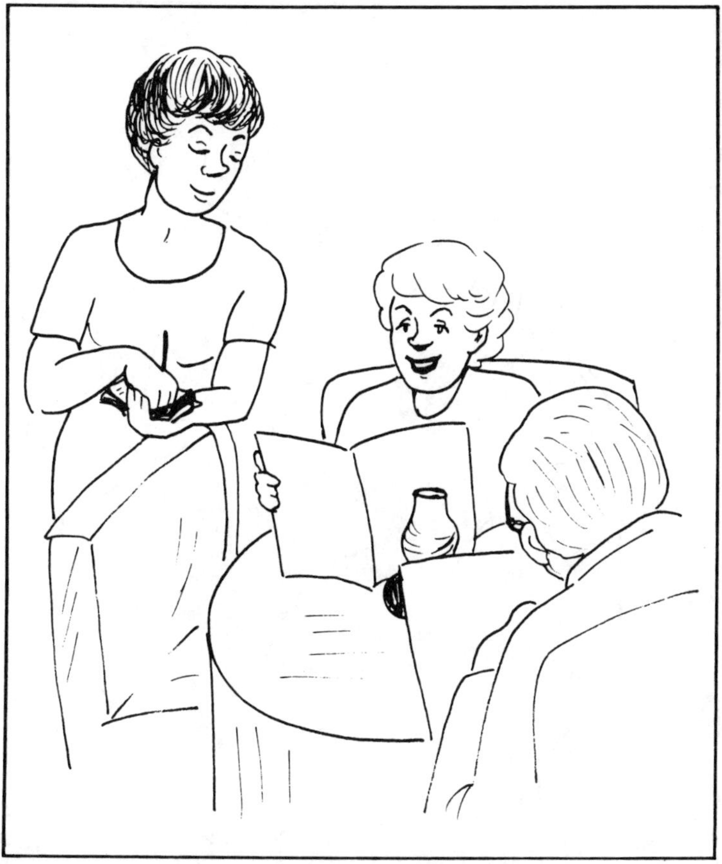

Fig. 3-7. The diabetic can eat out just like anyone else.

great problem once you've learned to select and balance foods off most menus (Fig. 3-7). You'll even be able to enjoy occasional desserts in moderation or fruits and cheeses.

The diabetic in control of his or her disease can travel with confidence. There are inexpensive travel kits that are safe and discrete to carry your injection materials. It is wise for the traveling diabetic to carry a small personal medical record with him containing any important health facts, as well as what medications and dosages have been prescribed in case another physician must be consulted in an emergency. A Medic-Alert bracelet can also be worn to warn any medical personnel of your condition in case you are incapacitated (Fig. 3-8).

In only the rarest of cases should diabetes prevent a person

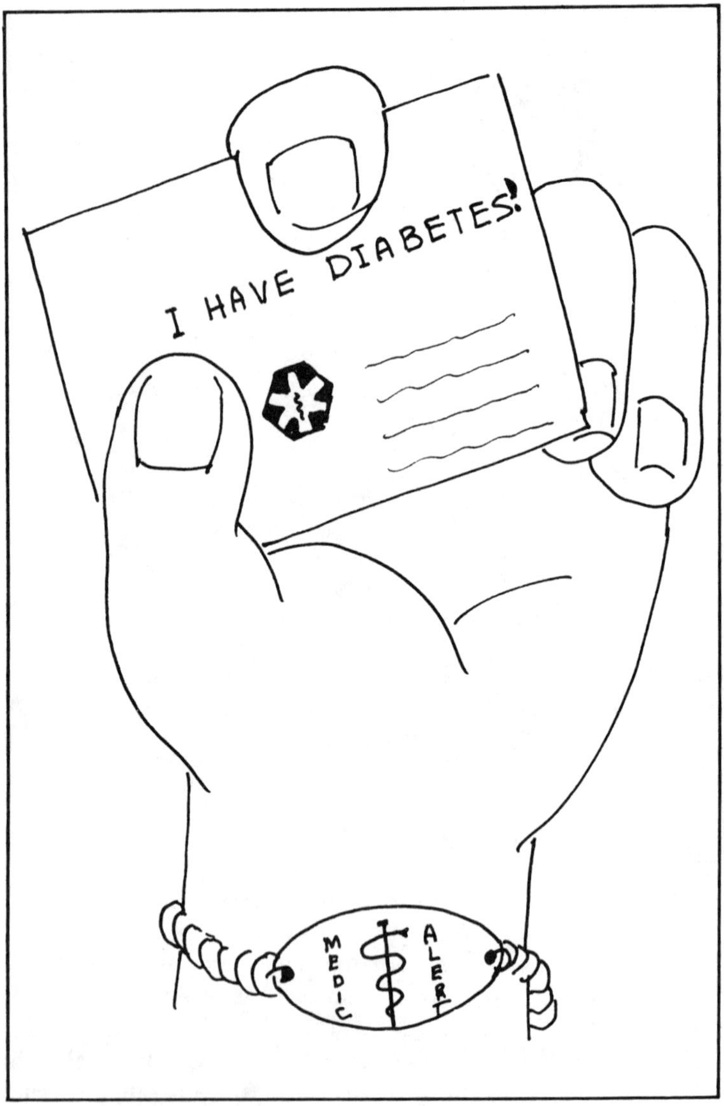

Fig. 3-8. Medical records and a Medic-Alert card and bracelet should be carried by the diabetic when traveling.

from marriage. It is important that you share as much information about your health with your intended spouse so that he or she can make rational decisions. There are a few instances where, due to circulation problems, male diabetics might have an impotence problem, but they are rare. If you suspect such a situation, discuss it frankly with both your physician and fiancee. Most women can have a normal pregnancy and normal children provided the physician knows of your diabetes and proper prenatal care is taken. Any diabetic woman considering marriage should, however, discuss the matter of pregnancy with her doctor and fiance openly and candidly.

The diabetic who is in control of his or her disease is little different from the non-diabetic and so can usually pursue the same life goals. Thus, coping with your diabetes means controlling your disease so that you can have a full and normal life.

4: Possible Complications

GOOD CONTROL OF YOUR DIABETES IS STRESSED TO AVOID THE possible complications of the disease. It is the complications that incapacitate the diabetic and prevent him or her from achieving a full, successful, and normal life. This chapter outlines some of the possible complications of diabetes, how to recognize them early, and what to do if you suspect any of the symptoms.

Your age has much to do with which complications you are likely to confront. Among young diabetics, kidney disease is most prevalent, while among adults it is rare. Adults, on the other hand, face problems stemming from circulation, which includes heart disease, stroke, arteriosclerosis, and visual problems. These are not frequent complications for the young diabetic.

CIRCULATORY PROBLEMS

All blood vessels are adversely affected by poorly controlled diabetes, especially the very smallest, the *capillaries*. It is the capillaries that carry blood to all the cells of the body. When the vessels are compromised by diabetic changes, they circulate less blood to the organs and muscles, denying them vital oxygen. In extreme cases diabetics may suffer gangrene. If you notice excessive bruising, slow healing of minor wounds, more than normal aching of muscles with even minor exertion, see your physician as soon as possible.

Heart Disease

Since the heart is the pump that circulates all the blood through the body, heart problems are also circulatory problems. Diabetics who do not maintain their blood sugars in good balance have a much higher incidence of heart disease. Heart failure and coronary heart disease are both serious and potentially deadly diseases which may be a consequence of poor diabetic control. If you are troubled with shortness of breath and/or chest pain with exertion, your doctor should be consulted immediately. If you tend to wake up at nights short of breath or have to sleep on several pillows to keep from gasping for air, you may be experiencing symptoms of congestive heart failure. All diabetics over 50 years old should have a cardiac evaluation every year as part of their physical examination.

Stroke

Stroke is also a problem of circulation. The brain is a remarkable computer that mediates everything we do and think. It requires a tremendous supply of energy which is derived from the blood circulating through it. If the flow of blood to a certain area of the brain is compromised, stroke may result. The symptoms of stroke vary greatly depending on which area of the brain is deprived of blood and oxygen. If it is a motor area, paralysis may result. In a speech area, the ability to communicate may be diminished or eradicated. Stroke can result from either a hemorrhage of a vessel or its blockage.

Diabetics who notice transient focal weaknesses, even brief memory lapses of increasing frequency, spells of disorientation, increasing periods of dozing off at inappropriate times, or periods of incoordination may be experiencing the warnings of an impending stroke. Immediate medical attention is indicated.

KIDNEY DISEASE

The kidneys are two small, bean-shaped organs, vital to life, which filter the entire blood supply of the body and withdraw impurities and waste products from it. These waste products are then discharged from your body in the form of urine. To accomplish their awesome task, these small organs filter the blood through small spheres, called *glomeruli.* These millions of microscopic glomeruli are surrounded by capillaries which allow the process of osmosis to clear the blood of its impurities. If your diabetes is allowed to go out of control for long periods of time, these vital and delicate tissues begin to leak. Vital proteins escape from the blood and some of the waste products are not filtered out. Renal failure and its consequences may result.

Diabetics who notice *edema,* or swelling, of ankles, legs, fingers, and other areas of the body due to fluid, should see their physicians. Another sign of renal problems is extreme fatigue without justifying activity. It may be due to the retention of waste products, known as *uremia.* Early medical intervention is necessary to avoid permanent, irreversible damage to the kidneys. Kidney disease is far more prevalent in the juvenile diabetic than in the adult-onset type.

HARDENING OF THE ARTERIES

Arteriosclerosis, or hardening of the arteries, is a normal part of the aging process. In the uncontrolled diabetic, this process is greatly accelerated. This disease may lead to heart disease, hypertension, stroke, kidney disease, blindness, or gangrene. Diabetics who have a tendency toward high blood pressure should be especially wary and insist on close medical supervision.

VISUAL PROBLEMS

Uncontrolled diabetes can lead to various eye problems. *Cataracts,* a cloudiness of the lens of the eye, and *glaucoma,* an increased pressure inside the eye which can cause blindness, are more prevalent in long-term diabetic patients. The main concern of diabetics, however, is, again, in the blood vessels.

Like circulatory problems in the rest of the body, the capillaries in the retina of the eye are subject to deterioration. The retina is the layer at the back of the eye which translates light impulses from the world around us into the chemical and electrical energy that becomes our sight. If the capillaries that supply the retina can no longer supply it with vital oxygen, the retina will deteriorate and so will the vision it mediates. Retinal detachment may occur.

Fortunately, medical progress has made it possible to save the sight of many who would have gone blind from this disease in the past, but early detection and intervention are essential.

Diabetics should have yearly eye examinations by qualified medical eye specialists. Diabetics who have difficulty maintaining their control should have eye exams at least twice a year.

NEUROLOGICAL PROBLEMS

Longstanding diabetes may cause deterioration of nerves in all

Table 4-1. Types of Coma & Their Differences.

Insulin Reaction or Coma	**Diabetic or Hyperglycemia** Reaction or Coma
EARLY SIGNS	EARLY SIGNS
Hunger	Drowsiness & Fatigue
Anxiety	Labored breathing
Headache	Energy loss
Heart pounding	Weakness
Heavy perspiration	Extreme thirst
Racing pulse	Increasing urination
Trembling	High amount of sugar in urine
Nausea	Slow onset
Rapid onset	Acetone (fruity) breath odor
Fainting	
Not able to awaken	
FIRST AID	FIRST AID
Give food with high sugar content if conscious. Do not force feed if unconscious.	Call a doctor
Give glucagon if unconscious.	Give insulin as directed by the doctor.
Call doctor.	Drink water. Do not force if unconscious.
Take to emergency room.	Test urine or blood frequently.
LIKELY CAUSES	LIKELY CAUSES
Overdose insulin	Too little insulin
Excessive activity	Over eating, too much sugar
Too little food	Infection, fever, stress
Delayed or missed meal	

areas of the body, especially in the extremities. These changes are usually irreversible by the time they are recognized, but fortunately they are rare in patients who have had their disease for less than 20 years. Good control of blood sugars drastically reduces the chances of neurological degeneration. Patients who suspect focal weaknesses, incoordinations, and intermittent but increasing numbnesses and pains, or unexplainable pains in their extremities should seek medical consultation.

COMA AND HYPERGLYCEMIA

There are two types of coma of which diabetics must be aware. One is caused by too much insulin, the other is from too little. They are known as insulin coma and diabetic or hyperglycemia coma respectively. Though the end result is similar, the onset and treatment are very different. Table 4-1 demonstrates the differences.

SUMMARY

Thinking about the possible complications to diabetes can be distressing, but remember that most diabetics do not experience these problems. The key to the avoidance of these problems is maintaining control of your disease.

A good rapport with your physician is essential. If you feel you have difficulty relating to your doctor or feel uneasy calling on him when you have worries or questions, consider changing doctors. If you have a good relationship with your doctor, then it is your responsibility to cooperate with him diligently. The final responsibility for controlling your diabetes is with you. No one else can make you follow the regimen that has been prescribed for you.

5: Deadly Habits

A FEW BUT VERY IMPORTANT WORDS MUST BE DEVOTED TO the subject of smoking, ingestion of excessive alcohol, and the use of narcotic drugs. These are dangerous habits for nondiabetics; they are deadly habits for diabetics. Furthermore, these substances are addicting. There is no question that smoking and alcoholism are drug addictions. Alcohol is three times as great a drug problem as all the "hard" drugs put together. Smoking is the number one public health problem in our nation.

If you have any of these habits, seek help to get rid of them. If you regularly ingest more than two or three alcoholic drinks a day you may have a drinking problem. If you doubt it, try to do without it for several days. If you can't stay away from alcohol, get professional help. It is a rare alcoholic who can kick the habit without help.

The same can be said of smoking. If you can't kick the habit cold turkey, get help to do it. The same goes for the use of marijuana, cocaine, or any other drug. Get help to rid yourself of any of these habits.

Alcohol, smoking, and drug abuse will potentiate your diabetes and speed the development of any or all of the possible complications to the disease. Smoking has a tremendously detrimental effect on your heart and circulatory system. It will cause elevation of your blood pressure and often leads to stroke.

Alcohol also is harmful to your heart, circulation, and central nervous system. In addition it is destructive to the pancreas and may destroy what little function you are getting from your beta cells.

Hard drugs damage your circulatory system and do irreversible damage to your central nervous system. Even prescription mind-altering drugs should be taken with great caution and only for brief periods of time. If you have been on a sedative, tranquilizer, or antidepressant medication for a long time, discuss it with your doctor before you become dependent on it.

It is important that you intervene in the use of any of these addicting substances before they do you more physical and mental harm. As a diabetic, they are far more dangerous to you. Do something about it now!

6: A Realistic, Hopeful Future

THE TECHNICAL PROGRESS OF THE PAST DECADES HAS literally given the diabetic a new lease on life. Prior to the advent of injectable insulin in 1926, diabetics had little to look forward to other than a future of suffering and fear. When the work of Dr. Frederick G. Banting, a young surgeon from Toronto, Canada, led to the successful extraction of insulin that could be injected into diabetics, all that changed. Since that time, knowledge and technical advances have made the fondest hopes of diabetics a reality. Life for most diabetics need be little different than for other people.

There is, however, even greater hope for the diabetic's future. Work is continuing in many areas to better understand the dynamics, physiology, and pathology of this disease. Pharmaceutical companies are working constantly to refine the armamentarium of medications available to the diabetic today, and to discover and develop newer and better drugs for the future.

Much work has already been done to develop medication delivery systems to eliminate human error. These are miniature computers programmed to discharge the exact quantity of medication into the diabetic's blood. They are so small they can be implanted into the body to work for months at a time. Developers of these electronic devices anticipate units that will "sense" the body's needs and adjust the dose to the exact needs of the patient as he or she alters activities. These electronic, computerized medication delivery systems are, in effect, miniaturized artificial pancreases.

Additional work is being done in the area of transplants, with the hope that healthy donor tissue will be reliably transplanted to replace nonfunctioning beta cells, virtually eliminating diabetes from the patient.

Research is constantly going on to understand the causes of diabetes and to perhaps discover a vaccine against infectious agents, such as viruses, that may be implicated in the disease. Other researchers are constantly seeking better ways to help patients cope with their diabetes. Educators are spreading the facts about diabetes, dispelling myths, and opening doors which have heretofore been closed to diabetics.

Simply put, diabetes is one of the diseases of man that is yielding to the efforts of science! Your future is truly bright with potential; but it is your responsibility to take advantage of it. You, your doctor, and your loved ones are a team pitted against a disease that is giving way. Make the best of your situation. Do not let your diabetes control you; take control of your health and your future!

Index

U

V

W

OTHER POPULAR TAB BOOKS OF INTEREST

44 Terrific Woodworking Plans & Projects (No. 1762—$12.50 paper; $21.95 hard)

How to Repair Briggs & Stratton Engines—2nd Edition (No. 1687—$8.95 paper; $15.95 hard)

Security for You and Your Home . . . A Complete Handbook (No. 1680—$17.50 paper; $29.95 hard)

46 Step-by-Step Wooden Toy Projects (No. 1675—$9.95 paper; $17.95 hard)

The Kite Building & Kite Flying Handbook, with 42 Kite Plans (No. 1669—$15.50 paper)

Building Better Beds (No. 1664—$14.50 paper; $19.95 hard)

Organic Vegetable Gardening (No. 1660—$16.50 paper; $25.95 hard)

The Woodturning Handbook, with Projects (No. 1655—$14.50 paper; $21.95 hard)

Clock Making for the Woodworker (No. 1648—$11.50 paper; $16.95 hard)

Steel Homes (No. 1641—$15.50 paper; $21.95 hard)

The Homeowner's Illustrated Guide to Concrete (No. 1626—$15.50 paper; $24.95 hard)

Kerosene Heaters (No. 1598—$10.25 paper; $16.95 hard)

Clocks—Construction, Maintenance and Repair (No. 1569—$13.50 paper; $18.95 hard)

The Underground Home Answer Book (No. 1562—$11.50 paper; $16.95 hard)

Airbrushing (No. 1555—$20.50 paper)

Basic Blueprint Reading for Practical Applications (No. 1546—$13.50 paper; $18.95 hard)

Central Heating and Air Conditioning Repair Guide—2nd Edition (No. 1520—$13.50 paper; $18.95 hard)

The Complete Book of Fences (No. 1508—$12.95 paper; $19.95 hard)

How to Sharpen Anything (No. 1463—$12.95 paper; $19.95 hard)

Building a Log Home from Scratch or Kit (No. 1458—$12.50 paper; $17.95 hard)

Build It with Plywood: 88 Furniture Projects (No. 1430—$13.50 paper; $18.95 hard)

The GIANT Book of Metalworking Projects (No. 1357—$12.95 paper; $19.95 hard)

The Welder's Bible (No. 1244—$13.95 paper)

The GIANT Handbook of Food-Preserving Basics (No. 1727—$13.50 paper; $17.95 hard)

Ventilation: Your Secret Key to an Energy-Efficient Home (No. 1681—$8.95 paper; $15.95 hard)

Tuning and Repairing Your Own Piano (No. 1678—$12.50 paper)

Superinsulated, Truss-Frame House Construction (No. 1674—$15.50 paper; $21.95 hard)

Raising Animals for Fun and Profit (No. 1666—$13.50 paper; $18.95 hard)

Practical Herb Gardening . . . with Recipes (No. 1661—$11.50 paper; $15.95 hard)

Effective Lighting for Home and Business (No. 1658—$13.50 paper; $18.95 hard)

Constructing and Maintaining Your Well and Septic System (No. 1654—$12.50 paper; $17.95 hard)

Maps and Compasses: A User's Handbook (No. 1644—$9.25 paper; $15.95 hard)

Woodcarving, with Projects (No. 1639—$11.50 paper; $16.95 hard)

Sign Carving (No. 1601—$13.50 paper; $19.95 hard)

Mastering Household Electrical Wiring (No. 1587—$13.50 paper; $19.95 hard)

Cave Exploring (No. 1566—$10.25 paper; $16.95 hard)

The Radio Control Hobbyist's Handbook (No. 1561—$19.50 paper)

Be Your Own Contractor: The Affordable Way to Home Ownership (No. 1554—$12.50 paper; $17.95 hard)

Beekeeping—An Illustrated Handbook (No. 1524—$10.95 paper; $15.95 hard)

101 Model Railroad Layouts (No. 1514—$11.50 paper; $17.95 hard)

53 Space-Saving, Built-In Furniture Projects (No. 1504—$17.50 paper)

The Home Brewer's Handbook (No. 1461—$10.25 paper; $16.95 hard)

Constructing Outdoor Furniture, with 99 Projects (No. 1454—$15.95 paper)

Draw Your Own House Plans (No. 1381—$14.50 paper)

The Fiberglass Repair & Construction Handbook (No. 1297—$11.50 paper; $17.95 hard)

TAB **TAB BOOKS Inc.**

Blue Ridge Summit, Pa. 17214

Send for FREE TAB Catalog describing over 750 current titles in print.